TWELVE PATHWAYS TO PERSONAL WELLNESS

An Activity Based Perspective for Wellness of Body, Mind and Spirit

DAVID M. ROGERS

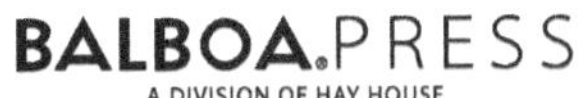

Balboa Press books may be ordered through booksellers or by contacting:

Balboa Press
A Division of Hay House
1663 Liberty Drive
Bloomington, IN 47403
www.balboapress.com
1 (877) 407-4847

Print information available on the last page.

ISBN: 978-1-9822-4251-0 (sc)
ISBN: 978-1-9822-4253-4 (hc)
ISBN: 978-1-9822-4252-7 (e)

Library of Congress Control Number: 2020902082

Balboa Press rev. date: 01/29/2020

CONTENTS

Introduction vii

Pathway #1 1
You are the One in Charge; You Control your State of Wellness.

Pathway #2 7
The Body was built to Move; Choose
Activities You will Perform Consistently.

Pathway #3 17
Fitness Requires a Combination of Aerobic,
Anaerobic and Flexibility Activities.

Pathway #4 23
Identify Your Body Type and understand your
Capabilities; Strive for Compatible Activities

Pathway #5 35
Create a Wellness Plan and Execute goals to sustain that Plan.

Pathway #6 51
Overall Balance is critical, in Wellness and in Life

Pathway #7 59
Variety is the Spice of Life and a Key to Wellness Also

Pathway #8 67
Garbage in Garbage Out; You Must
Properly Feed and Hydrate Your Machine.

Pathway #9 89
Rest and Recovery are an Important Part of Overall Wellness.

Pathway #10.. 97
Emotional Wellness; Attitude Influences Wellness Altitude.

Pathway #11 105
Nurture Your Positive Intellectual, Social, and Spiritual Passions

Pathway #12.. 113
Positive Renewal; Find Your Quiet Place

Appendix I – Financial Wellness Principles 119
Appendix II – Wellness from the Home to the Workplace 129
Afterword...141

INTRODUCTION

It was the late fall of my sophomore year in college. A fellow teammate had been begging me to visit a new fitness club that he wanted to join to maintain a daily off-season training regimen. To me, there was no such thing as off season training. We would go jogging once in a while or play a little tennis, soccer or touch football, but I thought there were better and less strenuous ways to spend the days ahead. My friend was persistent in his requests. I sensed that he might want me to support him as a work out partner. This was apparently not an adventure he wanted to undertake alone.

The day I walked through the door of the Berkley Fitness Center was a day that changed my life forever. The facility was located in a relatively cozy retail space in a local strip mall. As I entered the impeccably organized and maintained Center for the first time and looked around, I was met with a sight I had never seen before. A complete circuit of Nautilus® equipment was carefully arranged around the main room of the facility in a semi-circle. A small section of free weights occupied a distant corner. There were patrons working on the machines with a trainer at their side talking them through their movements and encouraging their performance.

We were met by the Fitness Center manager and given a tour of the facility. The machines fascinated me. Upon examining them more closely I could immediately sense the engineering, ergonomic integrity and cutting edge technology of each machine as the manager took us around the circuit and explained their program, how each machine worked and the Center's dedication to meeting our fitness expectations. I was intrigued. I had to try these captivating contraptions out. Within a few days I had become a member of the Fitness Center. Within a few weeks I was hooked.

One thing I quickly realized is that I did not have any expectations for what activities I needed or preferred. I did not have any goals. I really did not have any idea of general fitness principles. All I knew was that I enjoyed working on these futuristic looking machines. I had no idea how general physical fitness would transform over the following years into a lifelong philosophy of wellness. The type of wellness philosophy that promotes excellence and a desire for balance and achievement in every aspect of life. Nevertheless, that day was a transformational moment and I knew that daily, ongoing competitive exercise was going to become an integral part of my life. I also knew that I had a lot to learn.

Over the next few months and through the next few years my knowledge of fitness and the broader scope of wellness began to grow. The Fitness Center provided free personal training with my membership. And so I began my journey. Personal training sessions led to books on exercise methodology, health and nutrition. The Center offered fitness seminars with nationally renowned authors and trainers. Within a year I was invited to be an assistant manager of the center and personal trainer. Over these next several years, I enjoyed training and participating with fellow fitness enthusiasts, local high school and college athletes and corporate executives. I enjoyed this position until I graduated and left for a Master's program in another state.

Graduate studies opened broader horizons. Reading great authors of business, science, philosophy, religion, economics and other stimulating subjects opened to a young mind numerous doors, alluring pathways into a larger world. A more comprehensive life philosophy. A view of the universe that encouraged me to be my best. This is the foundation of lifelong wellness. Fitness came to mean more than a toned body. It encompassed soundness of mind and spirit. It transformed into a holistic view of being that embraced the fundamentals of overall wellness.

Fast forward several decades and the journey continues. I have been faithful to that initial transformational experience and have enjoyed a lifelong relationship with activity based wellness. The programs, places and faces have changed over the years, but the principles remain the same. Every individual has the opportunity to learn and benefit from incorporating proper wellness principles into their daily routine. Whether you have already had those transformational experiences or wish to step on the path to developing a personal philosophy of wellness the Pathways in this book will be timeless and priceless to a wellness based understanding of the whole self.

We live in an age where wellness programs abound. Gyms, holistic centers and specialized wellness facilities dot the landscape of every major city and suburb. Specialized routines that can be done at home are plentiful. The internet provides an almost unlimited stream of ideas and programs. Yet amidst this abundance of resources, the average person who commits to an activity based regimen of wellness usually does not stay with a program for more than sixty days. One of the main reasons for this is not necessarily motivational, it is a fundamental lack of understanding of the principles that sustain wellness. The Twelve Pathways will communicate those transformational principles in a simple and understandable manner.

A lifestyle of wellness is easier, more permanent and more complete if the underlying principles of wellness are understood and internalized. Interest in programs and pet philosophies may come and go, but an understanding of the Twelve Pathways ensures you will have the tools to be more consistently engaged. You will also be able to see and understand the positive progress of your own wellness journey. Whether we choose to recognize it or not, we are all governed by certain principles. Wellness has associated principles every bit as predictable and repeatable as simple gravity. The positive results you may achieve throughout your life will depend heavily on a respect for specific universal principles. In the chapters ahead we will explore these principles as outlined in the Twelve Pathways.

Wellness can be best defined as an overall completeness and soundness of being. Wellness assumes the incorporation of physical fitness into a framework that includes an equal balance of mental and spiritual capability. Wellness is generally viewed and defined as a healthy and balanced integration of the whole self, viewing the areas of mind, body and spirit as independently identifiable and sustainable parts of a greater whole. Wellness assumes application of beneficial principles in each of these areas, contributing to the fullest lifestyle possible in terms of overall health, enjoyment and achievement.

This book is not about specific programs or activities. It is about internalizing the underlying principles that can be applied to the myriad of programs and philosophies extant. Each Pathway contains a number of principles that, if understood, internalized and regularly utilized, will result in more complete and fulfilling personal wellness. They will change your life, and change it for the better.

No matter who you are, no matter what your circumstances, you can begin to become more proficient in all of these areas and increase your overall wellness starting today. The Twelve Pathways in this book are applicable no matter your age, weight, race, body type, gender or social status. The results these Pathways bring are consistently and universally applicable.

With the exception of overriding congenital or medical problems that might be constraining, everyone can undertake a journey that will bring greater strength and stamina, emotional and intellectual satisfaction and greater spiritual strength. Wellness engenders greater energy, clearer thoughts, and an increased ability to enjoy the positive things in life. Greater wellness just makes you…a better and more complete you!

As with all significant journeys, the journey to greater wellness begins one step at a time. Let's get started exploring the Twelve Pathways that will consistently improve and enhance your life.

YOU ARE THE ONE IN CHARGE; YOU CONTROL YOUR STATE OF WELLNESS.

Why consider wellness? If you ever heard the truism that wellness is a "state of mind" consider it as fact. But it is a fact that is linked to very real actions. The decision to form an ongoing dedication to wellness is a very personal one. It stems from recognizing that you have one life to live, one body to carry you through that life and one mind with which to navigate. The more thoroughly you maintain that whole being, strengthening and exercising every aspect of the body, mind and spirit, the more capable you will be to experience life's many joys and challenges.

A human being is a remarkable, complex and intriguing living system. There have been countless hours dedicated and funds spent throughout the years on researching, cataloging, identifying and understanding the various systems and functions of the human body. Yet, even at the rate new medical and scientific discoveries are being uncovered, we seem to have barely scratched the surface of the magnificent work of art and engineering that is a human being. The more closely we look at human existence, the more wonder and amazement we discover.

Personal wellness takes that combination of science and wonder and channels it into philosophical and behavioral specifics, geared to create and maintain the highest levels of health, fitness and mental performance. And that is an undertaking well worth your time, consideration and priority.

Amidst all of this wonder and discovery there is one universal, overriding principle that applies to anyone and everyone. That principle posits that you are personally in charge of how your body and mind are treated and maintained. You bear the ultimate responsibility for your health, intellectual development and overall well-being. While you may engage other people, places and services which can contribute to your wellness, you and you alone are accountable to carry through on a daily plan that leads you down the path of wellness. There are no substitutes, there are no shortcuts.

And so, the choice to learn and apply the principles of wellness, as illustrated in the Twelve Pathways in this book, is arguably the best and most necessary investment in yourself. You are the recipient of this investment in time and effort, as are all those with whom you are associated. They will benefit as well when you are at your best. And that is what wellness is always about, simply being your best. The day you decide to become accountable for your own wellness is the day you consistently implement the behaviors that reinforce this responsibility.

Hypertrophy versus Atrophy; the Human Entropic System

The first basic concept you must understand is that, as a biological system, your body is constantly in either a state of hypertrophy or atrophy. It is constantly subject to entropy, which dictates that without maintenance, it will systemically break down on a cellular level over time. This naturally occurs with age, but the decay of entropy can be slowed with proper application of wellness principles. It is key to understand the natural state of being demands constant attention and maintenance to keep systems from reverting to atrophy over time.

Whichever condition your body is in is solely dependent upon your decision and commitment to creating one state or the other. Hypertrophy is the state where the muscles, bones and circulatory systems of your body are growing stronger and more efficient. Maintaining hypertrophy means that your muscles are getting stronger, larger and denser. Your circulatory system is becoming more efficient at processing and distributing oxygen and nutrients to all areas of your body. Bone density and ligament strength are being reinforced. Brain activity is enhanced with more consistent oxygen and chemical levels.

In a state of atrophy, the opposite is happening. Your muscles are becoming smaller and less dense. Your other physical systems are becoming less efficient. Your cardiovascular health, the way your body processes oxygen and delivers essential nutrients through your blood, is in decline. Your brain will become deficient in certain nutrients and activity and will become duller.

The only difference between these two states of being is the choice to engage in activity that will result in hypertrophy. Such activities check entropy to an extent, extending the "youthful" activities and state of body and mind. That is, you must choose to undertake beneficial exercise and activities that will lead to a constant physical and mental state of hypertrophy.

The human body only takes a period of three to five days before it begins hypertrophy through continual exercise, or begins to atrophy due to lack of exercise. Lack of activity for only several weeks to a few months can result in a baseline of complete atrophy. In other words, to maintain hypertrophy, to maintain a level of continual or increasing wellness and health, you must constantly be engaged in beneficial movement and activity, which we generally call exercise. This is how the human body is encoded. This is how the body works. There is no way around this universal law of biophysics.

The same goes for your mind. Positive stimulation and activity have been shown to prevent mental decay. For example, a recent study by the National Academy of Sciences revealed that people who spoke a second language are protected from or delayed in the onset of Alzheimer's. The activity of learning and recalling keeps the mind growing on a neurological level.

The Argument for the Necessity of Physical and Mental Activity

Once you are clear on a basic understanding of how your body works and what activity levels are required to become and remain fit, it falls upon you to make the conscious decision to develop, execute and maintain a lifelong plan for physical activity. Research on the necessity of physical activity is plentiful. Study after study can be obtained and quoted, but they all come to essentially the same conclusion. If you exercise regularly, you will enjoy numerous benefits of increased health. If you do not exercise regularly you run a much higher propensity for numerous health risks.

In a twenty year study published in 1995 by then Surgeon General C. Everett Koop, some of the following benefits of sustained exercise were noted: greater physical stamina, clearer mental activity, greater memory retention, greater bone density and a decreased risk of osteoporosis, greater ability to maintain core body temperature, more efficient circulation, less risk of minor joint injury, less risk of coronary disease and so on. Conversely, lack of exercise has been listed in many studies to be linked to numerous health maladies including: obesity, diabetes, arteriosclerosis, increased risk of cancer, increased risk of heart disease or stroke, decreased bone density, increased risk of Alzheimer's and other mental deficiencies.

The results of decades of research are self-evident. Increased fitness, a primary cornerstone of overall wellness, means your life will be fuller and more productive. You will also look and feel better day to day with a daily regime of beneficial activity. But the decision still comes down to you. Your conscious decision to establish self-discipline, to learn the principles associated with effective types of exercise and to execute them will ultimately determine how far you will go and what degree of overall wellness you will experience.

In addition to physical movement in terms of exercise, stimulating the mind is also a significant part of wellness. Just as the body needs stimulation, so does the intellect. As we will discuss on subsequent Pathways, it is important to find activities that are mentally stimulating and challenge you to expand your intellect. This may come through working tasks, such as working with a second language or constantly running numerical calculations. But it mostly comes from extracurricular activities, such as reading, writing or creating art.

Whatever your choices for mental stimulation, you must keep your mind active. Long sessions on the couch in front of the television are not a healthy situation. Overuse of personal devices and gaming may actually have a deleterious effect on the mind. While some games, such as puzzles or word games, help exercise the brain, other games may actually set mentally acuity back in the brain, even reprogramming the attention span and creating other problems. Recent research has found significant correlation between using personal devices in excess to learning disabilities in primary and secondary aged children.

Other research is suggesting that serious addictions to tablets, phones and other devices in some subjects has stunted their social abilities. The designers of such devices have openly admitted that applications and programs are designed to provide dopamine hits to the brain similar to the ingestion of hallucinogenic drugs. While long term effects are still under study, the initial conclusions are not favorable.

Whatever the mental activity you choose, it should be both stimulating and fun. Like physical exercise, the most effective mental exercise is the type you will repeat often enough to sustain results. Constant stimulation is needed, but stimulation that is beneficial and keep the mind limber and powerful.

If you have already created a wellness oriented lifestyle, understanding and applying a consistent philosophy of mental and physical fitness will enhance and elevate that lifestyle. If you are still seeking to establish wellness as part of your daily life, make the commitment to learn and follow the proper fitness principles that will guide and change you. Resolve now to muster the discipline necessary to change yourself and enjoy your life to its fullest. The principles of activity oriented fitness are unfailing. The results are indisputable as an overall part of personal wellness.

Ultimately, it is up to you to make it all happen. It is a journey you CAN undertake. It is a journey you WILL undertake to be able to enjoy the richness and treasures a life of wellness has to offer you. You are responsible, and you can decide every day to maximize that responsibility!

Quick Tips to Control the State of your Wellness

- Create a personal fitness mission statement. Hang it in a place you will see it often.
- Sign up for a membership in a community fitness center. Make friends with like-minded individuals who are dedicated to fitness. Schedule concurrent workouts.
- Start a club for your favorite fitness activity in your community, e.g. biking, hiking or running club.
- Create a reward for doing so many days per week of exercise. For example: Five days of exercise earns a dinner out at your favorite restaurant.
- Create a blog about fitness. Share your successes and failures with others.
- Challenge yourself with fitness disciplines. For example: Ten days with no processed sugar in your diet. Reward yourself for achieving the challenge.
- Keep a log with pictures and detailed measurements that tracks the changes in your fitness levels and physique over time.

THE BODY WAS BUILT TO MOVE; CHOOSE ACTIVITIES YOU WILL PERFORM CONSISTENTLY.

The body was naturally built to move. The systems of the human body need movement and activity. To strengthen the muscles, joints and ligaments, to promote healthy cardiovascular function and to preserve a general sense of wellbeing. Precisely how the body moves is as individual as each of us. There are types of movement, regimens of exercise, which range from the highly competitive to the calming and contemplative. The daily activities of an individual that desires to exceed in a triathlon will look very different from someone who wishes to excel at yoga.

Both pursuits are worthwhile, and each may be the best fit for the individual undertaking them. And that is the point. The best exercise for you, the best way to get your body moving, is in a manner you decide is best suited for you that you will undertake consistently. Exercise that is not performed is simply not exercise. It may take some experimentation, but there is a "right" type of exercise for everyone. There has to be a desire, a connection and ultimately results that motivate you to keep moving. And move you must, or the effects of atrophy are waiting just a few days ahead.

Perhaps one of the most confusing and intimidating steps in embarking upon any fitness plan is determining which activities you will actually undertake. We live in an era where there is no shortage of facilities, equipment, programs or proponents of one method of exercise or another. There are innumerable ways to keep the body moving. The fitness industry in America is a multi-billion dollar business. You do not have to look far to come across a piece of fitness equipment or some program that makes claims to be the latest and greatest, easiest and most convenient or that promises the most immediate results.

The bottom line to achieving consistent physical fitness in an overall philosophy of wellness is simply this: the best exercise for you is that exercise that you find enjoyment and satisfaction in and that you will do repeatedly and consistently. To engage in frequent physical activity you almost certainly must find enjoyment in that activity and experience positive results from your efforts. For most individuals seeking higher levels of personal fitness, the process of finding that best exercise, or in many cases combinations of activities, is a journey often undertaken over time with periodic experimentation.

Your choices for regular fitness activities are numerous and may be a bit confusing with all of the claims that are being made. Whatever you choose to do, just remember to keep moving. Picture your journey into fitness activities similar to visiting a newly discovered restaurant district in a city near you. You will spend many evenings over several months visiting the various establishments and sampling their many dishes. You may have pre-conceived notions about how you like to dine. You may see yourself as a healthy eater and seek out the best salad bars. You may feel a preference for something more exotic, such as an appealing Oriental style of cooking or something from the Mediterranean. Inevitably you will settle in on a favorite place or two and tend to frequent them based on your tastes and desires for their specific menus. Preferences for exercise programs tend to evolve in a similar way.

It is not uncommon to embark upon an exercise routine based on the endorsement of others. Often it is a friend or trusted associate who communicates their passion and results from specific activities. Often there is a fitness community, such as a local gym, health club or wellness group at work that promotes activities that are attractive. Whatever the initial and ongoing attractors might be, the activities that you actually choose to embark upon and then remain engaged in over time are the best activities for you. Personal preference and those activities that resonate, feel good and bring positive results will be the most likely determinants.

Expectation Based Exercise and Performance

You will often pick exercise activities based upon some set of assumptions or perceived expectations. These expectations can be specifically goal oriented such as weight loss, improved muscle tone, increased stamina, etc. They can also be based on social expectations such as inclusion to a club, greater acceptance by peers, association with similar enthusiasts, etc. Whatever exercise you embark upon, realistically weigh the expectations you have for yourself.

For example, riding a bicycle for half an hour a day will not improve your upper body strength to a significant degree, although it might help with a weight loss goal. Perhaps training on a bicycle for half an hour a day could open doors to a local group that enjoys taking weekend bicycling trips into distant outdoor venues. Likewise, a modest jogging routine might help develop the stamina required to better enjoy skiing with a group of friends in the coming winter. You might select a resistance training program at a local gym with the expectation of building greater muscle mass. You might sign up for a cross training class to improve overall strength, stamina, flexibility and balance. Or you might take a company challenge to walk a certain amount of steps per day to obtain a personal or team reward.

Your performance of the activities you undertake should reflect the expectations that you have. If you are not seeing the results you desire you have only three choices. Increase the level of your current activity until you see results, choose a different activity that might better bring the desired results, or cease activity altogether. The third option should never be considered, even if it is often the choice when seeing a lack of results. You need to be flexible, open-minded and feel encouraged to try a different avenue if your expectations are not met by a specific activity. Remember, there are so many options available to you!

Whatever activities you embark upon, you will be more consistent and more successful if your expectations realistically reflect the goals and purposes you have envisioned. To truly achieve ongoing personal fitness, you will have to identify those favorite activities that you look forward to repeating on a regular basis. If your expectations of personal results and the associated applications and activities of exercise are realistic, you will be more satisfied and thus more consistent in pursuing those results.

Wellness is indeed a journey. And the goals of keeping your body in motion through personal fitness activities is a big and critical step in that journey. It is a journey you will be more eager to undertake if you find the going enjoyable and fulfilling. With activities that suit you, and that meet your expectations and help you experience positive results, it will continue to be a productive journey.

Activities that Fits Your Lifestyle

One major consideration of a wellness lifestyle is being able to integrate a schedule of activity compatible with a personal philosophy of fitness into the rest of the daily demands of life. Whatever activities you choose, it must find space in your lifestyle. The most common objection to consistent fitness activity is time. Convenience in many cases is essential. Quick and easy access to facilities, equipment or programs is a key criterion. If you are to make consistent fitness activity a goal, it has to take a reasonably high priority within the framework of other commitments. You have to assess the obstacles to fitness and find a way to overcome them on a daily basis.

Lifestyle can be harmonious or prohibitive in maintaining personal fitness. Whatever activities you choose must find a place within the current demands that you face. Many of the at-home programs that are flourishing today have taken the inconvenience of time into consideration. Whatever your demands, the chances are that you can find a program that fits within your lifestyle. With the average American watching over four hours of television per day, it seems likely that a minimum of fifteen to thirty minutes might be winnowed out somewhere to engage in fitness-improving activities. It boils down to a question of priorities. It begins with a determination of will. "Mind over mattress" and the will to make time whenever possible.

Making choices for fitness activities that fit within your daily schedule will eventually modify, enrich and change your overall lifestyle for the better. Fitness is indeed the cornerstone of greater overall wellness. Any investment in time or sacrifice of other priorities to include regular fitness activities will pay dividends in enriching other aspects of your life. Life is fuller and more enjoyable when a fitness plan is executed and you are experiencing the benefits of that plan. Fitness means an increase in physical energy and mental clarity for any other activities you may undertake including work, family and leisure. Personal fitness is a primary catalyst to transform your current lifestyle, incorporating active and wholesome priorities that define wellness.

Fitness and Life Phases

While the overall benefits of personal fitness activities can be realized at any age or any point in life, there are considerations that need to be recognized based on the phase of life you are in. The sad fact is that we do not remain twenty-five forever. The fitness activities that you may find most enjoyable at age twenty-five may not hold the same priority at age sixty-five. A personal fitness plan should evolve over time as you pass through the various phases of youth, middle age and elderly years. One of the joys of fitness based wellness is that there are productive activities that can be enjoyed at any age, assuming a general state of good health and lack of serious physical handicaps. But your choices in activities should be geared toward what is realistic and enjoyable given the phase of life you are currently in.

A fifty-five year old ex-football player with bad knees would probably be disappointed with setting a goal to run a marathon. A forty-five-year-old mother of three might find it constraining to try and set the same goals for a marathon and be better served to train for middle distance events. A sixty-five-year-old couple might find more satisfaction in swimming, hiking, bicycling, yoga or dance than they would in power lifting or rock climbing over thousand-foot high cliffs. Whatever your circumstances, there are activities that will enhance the phase of life you are in and prepare you more completely for the phases of life yet to come.

Activity levels for Youth and Young Adulthood, up to Age 35

The peak years of physical activity are obviously the younger years. Regardless of the sports, fitness, or other activities which take hold from youth up until roughly age 35, fitness is a blank slate, ready to be filled with any undertakings that catch your fancy. In youth and college-aged individuals, this may comprise specific sports and other activities. In early career phases, time may become a limiting factor as work begins and long hours may be the norm for many. These earlier years are a phase of life most opportune for developing a sustainable fitness based wellness philosophy. Habits developed earlier in life tend to benefit the middle and later years of life.

Even though this phase of life is a time where, assuming normal good health, you can eat almost anything and do almost anything, developing good habits and creating a foundation of fitness in a larger wellness lifestyle is crucial. It is much more difficult to begin and sustain fitness oriented programs as age increases. It is a much shorter climb from a sedentary lifestyle to an active lifestyle in younger years. The physical entry barriers are considerably easier.

Activities in this period of life can encompass almost anything. From running road races, to playing professional sports, to attending aerobics classes to participation in a CrossFit group. You may set a goal to hike the Adirondacks or ski every resort in California. Any of these activities are available depending on your situation. You will be able with consistent activity to achieve almost any reasonable fitness goal you may have.

The one caution to youthful enthusiasm in such activities is the risk of overdoing it. For the notably gung-ho fitness enthusiast, injury is the one occurrence that can derail the fun. This is a time of life where enthusiasts seek to stretch themselves, looking for the next level of accomplishment. But stretch reasonably and with wisdom. Extreme overuse can bring injury, temporary or permanent. Enjoy and accomplish, but use reasonable discretion.

Activities for Middle Age, Ages 36-65

Middle age is a time of transition. It is a period when the entropic systems of the body start to edge in on fitness levels. This is not to say that an overall philosophy of wellness needs to change during this period. It simply means that as the middle age years roll on, it is wise to make adjustments.

One of the great problems as we progress through middle age is that we emotionally feel that we can physically sustain activities similar to our younger years, yet our bodies are beginning to slow. To quote the famous phrase "Our mind is writing checks our body can't cash". If you are active in this age group you will understand the need for lessening impact and longer recovery from vigorous activities.

As the years add up, it is a natural phenomenon to require less strenuous activity and longer recovery times. As we will discuss later, recovery time is almost important as the activities which require that recovery. Middle age is a time of adjustment. The volume and intensity of whichever activities you prefer need to be adjusted to levels your body can reasonably sustain.

This may be a phase of life where long distance running gives way to less impactful middle distance running, or long distance cycling. Power lifting might yield to circuit training. Hiking tall mountains might segue into hiking long rolling trails. One constant will be to gradually decrease the impact and wear on the body as years and decades roll on. Unlike earlier years, the sense of invincibility may give way to a more realistic and sustainable perspective of what constitutes beneficial activity.

In this phase of life, accumulation of experience and wisdom compensate for gradual physical decline. We tend to find a more natural balance of self as we progress through these years. Barring an unusual need for competitiveness, it is a natural process to "ease off the gas" a bit and adjust activity levels to the levels of stress appropriate with your effective age. But the goal is to keep moving. It is simply the quality and quantity of movement that should be shaped to the demands of time and aging.

Activities for Senior years, Age 66 and up

The later years in life provide numerous and continued opportunities to integrate fitness into an overall lifestyle of wellness. One of the great benefits of this phase of life is a long tenure of experience. You know what you like and do not like. You have a solid idea of what works and what does not. But, as with any other time in life, the objective is to keep moving.

While this phase of life is a difficult time to begin a strenuous fitness regime, it can be done but must be undertaken carefully and gradually. If you have built a foundation of fitness through the years, the main goal in this phase is to maintain fitness levels as consistently as possible. This is not a time for massive fitness gains. It is a time for gently sustained fitness goals.

If career responsibilities are lessened at this point, there is more time to focus on overall wellness goals and activities. The more esoteric intellectual and spiritual pursuits may take precedence over physical activity. But fitness activity should not be neglected or abandoned. Sociality and like-minded individuals are a great resource in this phase. It is a time of life where it is even more fun to be active together.

The golden years can indeed be golden for wellness. If you continue to be active in this phase you can reap the dividends of years of wellness. You can enjoy a longer, fuller and more meaningful senior season. There are no absolute scientific guarantees to a longer life, even with a comprehensive approach to wellness (although recent studies are suggesting certain health practices may contribute to greater longevity) but continued wellness promises a much richer quality of life in the senior years.

As in other phases, the key is to keep moving, keep active. It is also important to continue to identify activities that have intrinsic meaning and reinforce your value system. Keeping your mental and spiritual activities moving are especially important in this phase of life. Do what you love; love what you do!

Quick Tips for Choosing the Best and Most Consistent Activities

- Search the Internet for various fitness programs. Read and study the program details and claims of each.
- Join a local gym on a short term membership. Sign up for personal training and ask for a trainer that can take you through a variety of routines.
- Network with friends or colleagues who are into fitness. Discuss what they are doing and find out what works for them and what sounds interesting to you.
- Keep a journal of your fitness progress. Record what exercise you enjoyed, what gave the best results and identify those activities you enjoying doing most frequently.
- Resolve to try one new activity per month, for example take a dance class, a Pilates class, purchase an exercise DVD, or plan a new biking or running route.
- Experiment with high impact exercise such as running or weight training. Then as a contrast experiment with low impact exercise such as yoga. Test how each makes you feel.
- Have a friend join you as a workout partner. Take turns challenging each other once a month to embark on a new exercise adventure together.

FITNESS REQUIRES A COMBINATION OF AEROBIC, ANAEROBIC AND FLEXIBILITY ACTIVITIES.

The concept of fitness, as it harmonizes with a philosophy of complete wellness, involves constant physical activity. Those activities can be broken down into specific types of activity, which have a specific effect on the body. A combination of these activities is recommended for effective overall fitness. Each is necessary for the balance needed to help your body function at its best. These activities can be subdivided into aerobic activities, anaerobic activities and flexibility activities. These will each be explained more thoroughly below.

A tremendous body of research exists that delineates exactly what the human body responds to in terms of exercise. The highest levels of fitness are achieved when the human body is stressed in certain productive ways and recovers from that stress with increased strength, flexibility and cardiovascular efficiency. As discussed in Pathway #1, you are only three to five days away from increasing your fitness levels through activity, or having fitness levels begin to erode due to inactivity.

Activities that you choose to become involved in should incorporate each of the following: aerobic training to increase your cardiovascular endurance; anaerobic activities that incorporate some form of resistance training; flexibility exercises that keep muscles, ligaments and tendons supple and free-moving. Whatever programs or activities you enjoy, your optimum levels of personal fitness will be achieved when you incorporate all three of these aspects into your routine.

Aerobic Activity

Aerobic activity consists of activities that will raise your heart rate and respiratory rate to a certain level for a sustained period of time. There are numerous studies that outline safe and sustainable criteria for appropriate elevated heart rates. The range for aerobic activity is generally agreed to be 60% to 80% of your maximum heart rate based on your current age. The key to this principle is that the activities you choose should incorporate regular sustained aerobic activity at a level that is comfortable while still yielding improved cardiovascular benefits.

Generally accepted standards for minimal aerobic activity have been established at fifteen minutes of sustained activity at least three days per week. As with most physical activity, the more, the merrier up to the point that your body can endure regular activity without severe discomfort, and does not push far past a point of diminishing returns in terms of recovery. The most important muscle in the human body is the heart. Regular aerobic activity has been directly associated with a healthy heart and is linked to prevention of heart disease. Working your heart and lungs aerobically yields tremendous benefits to stamina and cardiovascular efficiency, as well as to increased mental clarity.

Examples of popular aerobic activities include walking, hiking, jogging, bicycling, dancing, cross-fit training, traditional aerobics classes, cross country skiing, circuit training and swimming. Any activity that involves the movement of large groups of muscles for sustained periods, leading to increased heart and respiratory rates sustained over a period of at least fifteen minutes should bring positive results. The best aerobic activity for you is the one you will enjoy the most and perform on a regular basis.

Anaerobic Activity

Anaerobic exercise is defined by short bursts of exertion, usually less than one to one and a half minutes in length. Resistance is usually involved in anaerobic activity. Resistance training occurs when a muscle or group of muscles exerts force against another object or against gravity. Anaerobic activity uses up your muscle's capacity quickly, resulting in rapid fatigue in the direction of resistance. Anaerobic activity yields minor cardiovascular benefits, but is directed more specifically at increasing strength and muscle mass.

Resistance training has evolved as a more specific discipline only in the last several decades. As late as the 1980s there were still numerous myths surrounding traditional resistance and strength training. Misleading ideas of losing athletic prowess due to muscle-bound, inflexible growth abounded. It was long thought that women could gain no benefit whatsoever from anaerobic strength training. Modern research in exercise physiology has shown these myths to be false. Anaerobic training, done properly, actually increases flexibility. Increased muscle mass has numerous benefits, including aiding in endurance, mental acuity, maintaining core temperature and resistance to disease and illness. Muscle mass is also the key component of the body that consumes calories and fuels a vigorous metabolism, key factors in reducing body fat and preventing unwanted weight gain.

Traditional examples of anaerobic activity include pull-ups, push-ups, sit-ups, weight training, rock climbing, power lifting, plyometrics, sprinting, gymnastics and other activities that provide brief and intense resistance. Anaerobic resistance activities should be done at least three times per week and in a manner that involves all of the major muscle groups of the body. Balance and working through full ranges of motion are more crucial criterion when training for strength than in aerobic activities. This will be discussed further in Pathway #6.

Strength and endurance are the combined cornerstones of overall personal fitness. A body with a healthy combination of muscle mass and cardiovascular efficiency is a body well prepared for any of life's challenges. But there is one other consideration that needs to be addressed.

Flexibility Activities

The concept of balanced overall of fitness would not be complete without covering activities that develop and maintain flexibility. Flexibility is best described as being able to move your muscles and joints comfortably through their fullest range of motion. Flexibility maintains muscle smoothness, proper muscle density and overall balance. Flexibility is important to sustain proper interaction between muscles and the joints and ligaments that unite your musculoskeletal structure. Maintaining flexibility is necessary to prevent injury to muscles or joints. If your muscles and joints are limber and flexible, you will be more comfortable whether active or sedentary. Flexibility exercises are often the most overlooked aspect of fitness. Flexibility can be maintained by traditional stretching exercises, yoga and certain types of massage therapy.

When it comes to complete fitness, evaluate the programs you engage in, or wish to commence. Do your activities accommodate all three of these concepts? If not, what might you need to do to ensure you are experiencing benefits in all three of these areas? As you formulate a philosophy of wellness, these are important technical considerations that should define the appropriate activities you undertake. You will achieve a more complete state of wellness if your body has been worked effectively in all of these areas.

Quick Tips for Total Body Fitness Activities

- Keep a journal of your fitness routines. Identify what mixture of aerobic, anaerobic and flexibility routines you do in a given week. Evaluate in terms of overall fitness goals.

- Make sure you are getting at least three fifteen minute aerobics sessions per week.
- Test your flexibility monthly with a pre-established set of stretches. For example, can you stretch and touch your knees, your ankles, your toes, palms to the floor, etc.
- Review your routines with a friend, colleague or exercise professional. Review your routine and log suggestions for greater balance among the various core activities.
- Employ a fitness expert, such as a personal trainer or wellness coach. Review your activities and evaluate in terms of the three areas of fitness.

IDENTIFY YOUR BODY TYPE AND UNDERSTAND YOUR CAPABILITIES; STRIVE FOR COMPATIBLE ACTIVITIES

We live in an era of mass media, a media that contains a number of inaccurate or idealized portrayals and messages. It is impossible to avoid athletes, celebrities and other icons that are represented as examples of physical perfection. It is impossible to count the number of people and programs that have been inspired by such examples. However, reality hits hard when a fitness program does not change the new enthusiasts reflection in the mirror into something closely resembling their expected idyll.

A very common reason that individuals fail to stay with a fitness centered ideology of wellness is a misunderstood or misguided view of what they can ultimately physically achieve. The vision they initially entertain of themselves somehow is not translated into reality. Comparisons with examples of other physiques that may or may not resemble the ultimate capabilities of your personal physical potential are generally more discouraging than helpful. An underlying reason for this may stem from a misunderstanding of basic physiology.

We are all born with a certain combination of genetic possibilities. In essence, we have to "play the hand we are dealt" when it comes to our ultimate physical goals and possibilities. You cannot change the genetic formula you have been given from birth, you can only take what you have and make it the best it can possibly be.

Years of research and study on the human anatomy have resulted in three basic classifications that describe body type. These classifications are important to understand in that each classification tends to respond to different activities in slightly unique ways. Knowing your body type, or at least being able to place your physical constitution within a general framework of classification will aid you in planning and executing the best activities for your particular body type. The more your preferred activities cater to your body's strengths, the more quickly you will experience positive results and remain dedicated to a course of sustained fitness activity.

The three main classifications that are generally referred to in anatomical literature are Ectomorph, Mesomorph and Endomorph. These classifications of human physical shape, referred to as somatotypes, are also known as the Sheldon Classification System. While each somatotype suggests a general description of predominant physical tendencies, it is rare that an individual matches only the characteristics of one body type.

Most people lean predominantly towards one of the types, but may also have a few characteristics of one or both of the other types as well. We are all somewhat unique in the mixture of genetic tendencies we inherit from our parents. A key to activating your highest levels of personal fitness involves accurately identifying what body type you possess and engaging in activities that best match your body's capabilities and tendencies. The three body types are illustrated below:

SOMATOTYPES

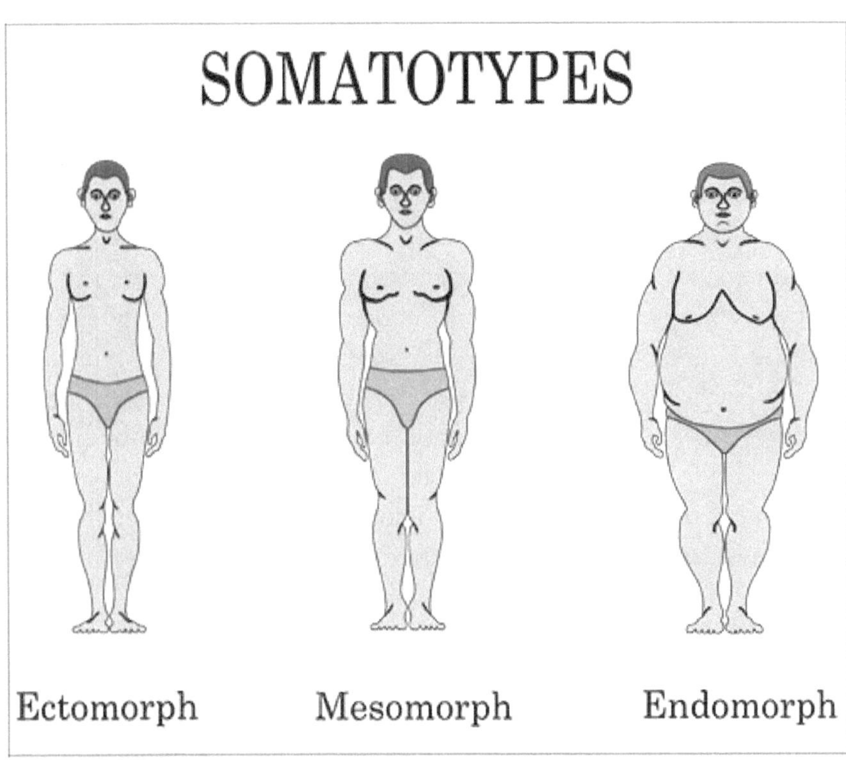

As outlined in Pathway #2, the best activities are those you will enjoy, that yield positive results and that are sustained over time. You have a much better chance of identifying activities that will bring you positive results if you understand your body type and cater to the unique needs of that body type. The three main somatotypes are discussed below.

In your personal assessment of body type, be realistic. It does not help to yearn for a different body type than you were born with. What is most important is that you do the best with what you are given. Over time, being honest and learning about yourself, including your body composition, what makes you happy and what gives you the best personal results, will ultimately lead to the most personal satisfaction. Personal wellness revolves around becoming comfortable with who you really are and what your inherent capabilities make possible.

<u>Ectomorph</u>

The ectomorphic body type is lean and slender with a light build. The overall physique is narrow with shoulder width not much greater than hip and torso width. The tendency is towards a linear physique from head to toe. Bone structure is light, joints are narrow and musculature tends to be light and lean. Ectomorphs tend not to carry much body fat and with proper training maintain low body fat over time. The chest and rib cage tends to be narrow also, often with a fairly long torso lending to above average height. Arms and legs are generally longer than average and tend to be very slender with light muscle mass. Facial structure tends towards tall and thin, with a high forehead and narrow cheeks and a long pronounced nose. The chin is often recessed. Ectomorphic musculature overall is light and consists of thin, lean muscle fiber.

Ectomorphic body types are predisposed to more endurance-oriented exercises. Ectomorphs tend to have larger proportions of white, slow twitch muscle fiber. This gives Ectomorphs the ability to excel at endurance-oriented activities. It takes more effort for Ectomorphs to build muscle mass, which can often be a slow and unrewarding undertaking for many individuals who possess this build type but hope for a more muscular physique. It is not uncommon for extreme Ectomorphs to gain only a few pounds of muscle per year even with significant resistance training.

Suggested exercises for Ectomorphs: hiking, biking, medium to long distance running, aerobics, circuit training, triathlons, cross country skiing, martial arts, cross-fit training, swimming, basketball, tennis, soccer and dancing.

Notable Individuals with Predominantly Ectomorph Somatotypes: Jon Heder, Bruce Lee, Eddie Murphy, Chris Tucker, Robert Pattinson, Kevin Durant, Randy Moss, Nicole Kidman, Cameron Diaz, Gwyneth Paltrow, Uma Thurman, Lisa Leslie and Jessica Ennis.

Mesomorph

Perhaps the most envied body type is that of the Mesomorph. This is the classic body builder physique that features a thick and broad skeletal system with broad shoulders, a large chest and narrow waist. The arms and legs are heavily muscled with pronounced muscular size and definition. The head and neck tend to be broad, square and thick. The Mesomorph also tends to carry low levels of body fat. Sedentary Mesomorphs can add body fat easily but are able to shed it more easily once consistent exercise is undertaken.

Joints are thick and strong, and the Mesomorph carries a higher percentage of fast twitch muscle fiber. Mesomorphs have a tendency to gain muscular power and strength rapidly with exercise and can increase muscle mass with relative ease. The only weakness to a Mesomorphic build is the tendency to struggle at more endurance oriented activities. Although with proper training, Mesomorphs can develop substantial endurance as well as power.

Suggested exercises for Ectomorphs: Power lifting, weight lifting, football, sprinting, shot-put, boxing, wrestling, martial arts, rugby, plyometrics, rock climbing, downhill skiing, and swimming.

Notable Individuals with Predominantly Mesomorph Somatotypes: Sylvester Stallone, Arnold Schwarzenegger, Duane Johnson, Karl Malone, LeBron James, Herschel Walker, Terrell Owens, Mark Wahlberg, Vin Diesel, Brittany Spears, Jessica Biels, Carmelita Jeter, Halle Berry and Madonna.

Endomorph

The Endomorph is a body type that is primarily defined by softness and roundness. Endomorphs have a round head and a thick and often short neck. Their torso is defined by a round abdomen, with arms and legs that are short relative to their overall height. Endomorphs carry greater than average to excessive amounts of body fat. They can gain and retain body fat easily. Endomorphs have large arms and legs that taper towards the wrists and ankles. Their feet and hands tend to be smaller than average.

Endomorphs tend to have a large ribcage with large organs, especially the stomach and heart. Endomorphs can gain muscle mass and strength from exercise fairly readily, but their muscular definition tends to remain masked under layers of body fat. Endomorphs appear wide relative to their height from side to side and from front to back. Their shoulder, chest and waist measurements remain fairly close and uniform.

Endomorphs can be divided into two basic sub-types also. There is the "apple" body shape that tends to carry a larger proportion of body fat in the upper body, particularly the chest, back and abdomen. A second sub-type is described as the "pear" body shape. This shape tends to carry more proportional fat in the waist, hips and legs as opposed to the upper body. Endomorphs face more difficult challenges in maintaining high fitness levels and keeping overall body mass within healthy parameters. But they can respond positively to consistent and proper exercise and nutrition.

Suggested exercises for Endomorphs: swimming, aqua-aerobics, bicycling, rowing, circuit training, weight lifting, aerobic dancing, hiking, walking and yoga.

Notable Individuals with Predominantly Endomorph Somatotypes: Jonah Hill, Jack Black, Kevin James, Seth Rogen, Charles Barkley, Mike Golic, Danny DeVito, John Goodman, Oprah Winfrey, Jennifer Lopez, Roseanne Barr, Christina Hendricks and Queen Latifah.

Understanding White and Red Muscle Fiber

In addition to the basic somatotypes, it is important to understand the two fundamental types of muscle fiber. Your body type will ultimately determine the amount and type of each muscle fiber you have available for physical activity. Muscle fibers can be broken down into two categories: white, or "slow twitch" muscle fiber and red or "fast twitch" muscle fiber. Red fibers have two sub-types known as intermediate and fast twitch fibers, but for the purposes of this discussion we will label them all fast twitch. Each body type suggests a slightly different distribution of these types of muscle fibers. The percentage of fast twitch and slow twitch muscle fibers you are genetically gifted with play a huge role in what exercises will benefit you the most.

White or slow twitch muscle fibers fire more slowly and are more efficient at using oxygen to burn the chemical fuel that fires your muscles. Therefore, they can operate over longer periods of time and fatigue much less quickly. Slow twitch muscles, when properly trained, can fire for hours on end without fatigue.

A predominance of slow twitch fibers suggests that you would excel at endurance events such as a marathon or triathlon. Top level marathoners have been analyzed as having up to 80% of their musculature composed of slow twitch muscles. Consequently, a predominance of slow twitch muscles also suggests it would be hard to pack on a large amount of muscle mass. Slow twitch fibers do not grow rapidly, therefore resist extreme hypertrophy that short-burst power exercises would stimulate.

Red or fast twitch muscle fibers have a faster rate of contraction than slow twitch, burn energy much more rapidly and fatigue quickly. But they are also capable of generating more powerful bursts of strength and speed. Training for fast twitch muscle fibers consists of short and explosive exercises such as weightlifting, sprinting or plyometrics. Fast twitch muscle fibers are capable of more rapid hypertrophy, contributing to muscular size and definition.

Research is ongoing to determine whether or not training can alter the combination of red and white fibers throughout our physiology. It has long been believed that we are born with certain proportions of muscle fiber and those proportions remain steady throughout our lives. Modern nutrition and training techniques are seeking to see if the formula within an individual can be altered but there are no universally agreed upon results to date. Again, it is best to assume for a personal fitness philosophy that you should play to your strengths versus trying to alter your basic physiology.

Somatotype Diagram

As mentioned earlier, most people do not meet all of the criteria of each somatotype precisely, but are somewhere along a continuum of characteristics from two or more somatotypes. A careful analysis of your own physiology, perhaps with some professional tools of analysis, can more accurately classify your specific physiology. A basic diagram showing the somatotypes is illustrated below:

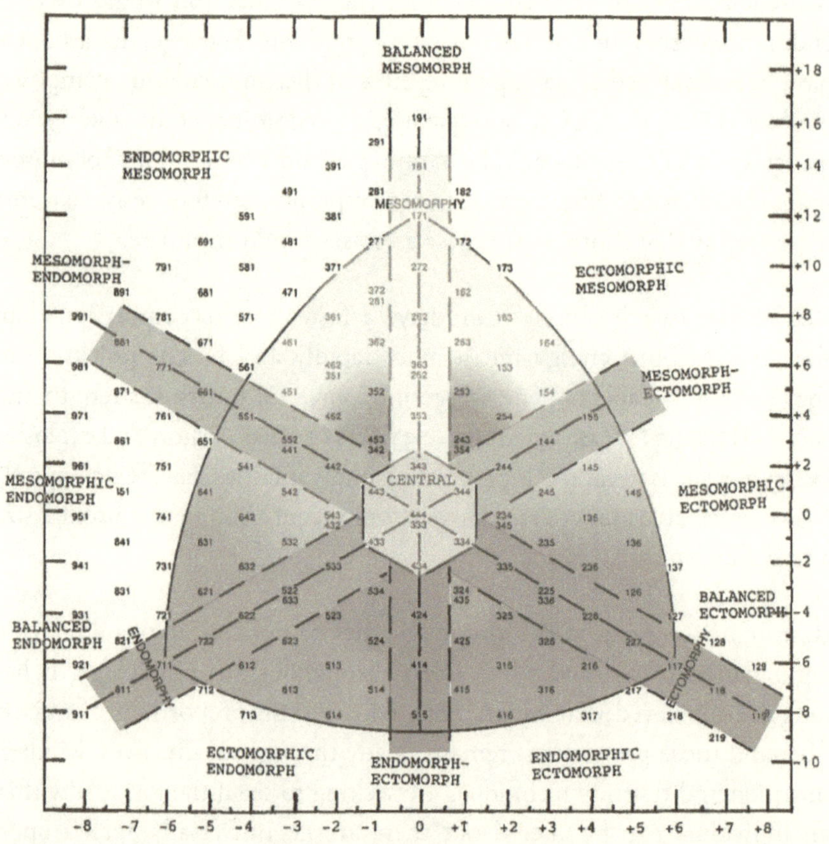

Body Somatotype Diagram

Every body type falls somewhere within this continuum. Again, the key is to understand your basic physiology and play to the strengths that your own unique physiology suggests. By taking this step you will trend toward more realistic goals and activities that will sustain your fitness and wellness over time.

Body Type and Body Mass Index (BMI)

A current standard for determining if your size and weight are within generally accepted health guidelines is known as the Body Mass Index (BMI). The BMI takes a measurement of your height and weight and establishes a scale to determine if these measurements are within healthy parameters. For the U.S. system in inches and pounds the formula for BMI = *mass(lbs)/height(in)2 x 703*. Generally, a BMI between 18 and 25 is considered optimum body weight while a BMI of 30 is considered obese and a BMI of 40 is morbidly obese.

As a general guideline BMI is a reasonable yardstick to assess your general size and weight in relation to a goal of overall wellness. However, the BMI does not take into account body composition and should therefore not be thought of as a hard and fast rule. Different body types have different proportions of muscle and fat. A key to wellness based fitness is to idealize muscle mass and muscle potential for use in your preferred activities. It is also a primary goal to minimize excess body fat. Depending on your body type and gender, the ratios may or may not fit squarely within the BMI as currently constituted.

For example, an individual very dedicated to strength training that is 5'11"and weighs 220 pounds has a BMI of 33 and is considered obese based strictly on standard BMI charts. However, if that weight consists mainly of muscle mass and the individual only has 10% body fat, they are certainly not obese but have in fact achieved a high level of hypertrophy and fitness.

Conversely, an individual that is the same height and weighs 175 pounds but has 32% body fat, though their BMI is only 24, should reconsider their fitness and training activities. A marathon runner that is 5'11 and weighs

135 pounds is considered underweight with a BMI of 17. However, this might be an ideal competition weight for such an individual based on their actual experience.

Illustrated below is a standard BMI chart. Remember that BMI is a useful guideline, but should be regarded as flexible based on your body type and overall wellness goals.

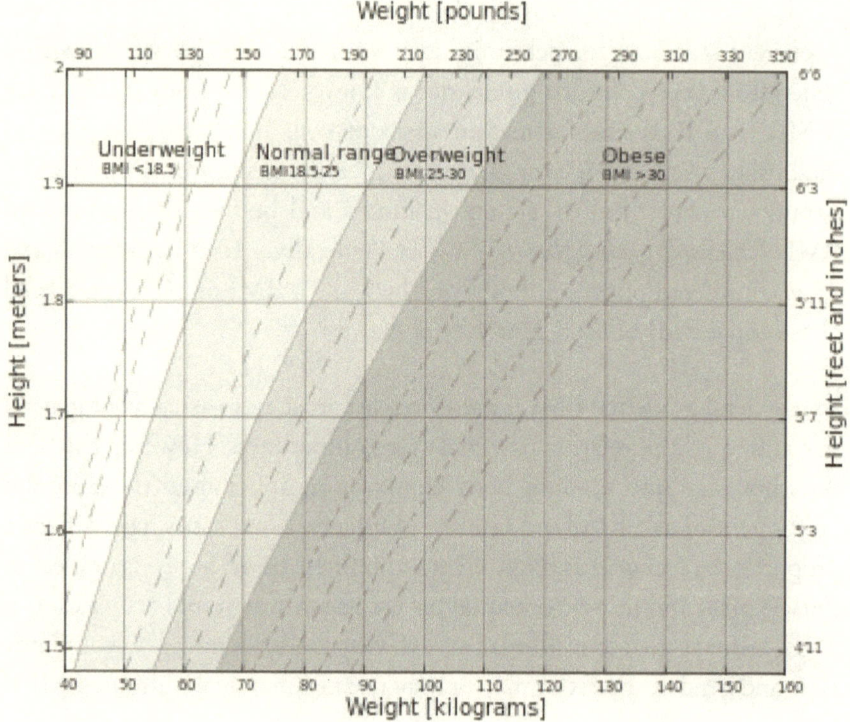

Quick Tips for Understanding Your Body Type and Planning Compatible Activities

- Undergo a professional Body Composition Analysis. Based on your total composition establish strength and endurance goals and activities.
- Gather images of well-known individuals that have similar body types. Identify strengths and weaknesses of your respective body

types. Compile a plan to play to the strengths and avoid the weaknesses.

- Make a list of goals for your specific body type. Identify specific targets, e.g. lower body fat by x percent, increase bench press by x pounds, run two miles in under xx minutes.
- Identify friends and colleagues with similar body types. Find out what they are doing that is working for them. Plan joint fitness activities together.

CREATE A WELLNESS PLAN AND EXECUTE GOALS TO SUSTAIN THAT PLAN.

Sustained wellness over time becomes more than a daily routine, a certain set of exercises or specific activities. It becomes a state of mind. Your personal vision of wellness may change over time depending on your age, understanding and experience. It is relatively easy to stay physically fit at age twenty-five. However, you have to pay more attention to the details if you are embarking on regular fitness activities for the first time in your forties. If you are age sixty, there are even more physical considerations to creating and maintaining a wellness plan.

At age twenty five, advanced mental pursuits or spiritual undertakings may be down on the priority list. At age sixty five, a much more metaphysical view of life and meaning tends to occupy our thoughts. But no matter what your stage of life, no matter what your physical or intellectual makeup, no matter how dedicated you have or have not been in the past, you must have a vision, a plan, and set certain goals that define your overall philosophy of wellness. A wish not quantified or written down remains a wish forevermore. A wish written down or designed into a plan becomes a goal.

However you feel about planning and goal-making, remember that wellness will always be a personal responsibility and a personal choice. It must be a way of life you choose and become dedicated to if you are to be successful. You have one life to live. You will live it as mentally, spiritually and physically fit as possible, or you will not. Whatever your goals in life, you will live them more enthusiastically and more fully within a philosophy of fitness based wellness than you would otherwise. The stronger your body and mind, the more capable you are of accomplishing whatever you set out to do. Your vision of yourself and the goals and plans you make will be more complete in the context of overall wellness. Your internalization of wellness reflects a fuller and well-lived life.

Your Personal Vision

What is it you inevitably see yourself becoming? What does a completely balanced and healthy you look like, act like and feel like? What are the main priorities that define your own wellness? Where do you want to see yourself in a month, in six months, in a year, in ten years? Have you seriously sat down and thought through a vision of your best self? Is your vision realistic? Have you an idea of what sort of commitment and dedication will be required to realize that vision? Are you willing to develop a principle based plan and put it into motion on a daily basis? Are you willing to hold yourself accountable to whatever plans or programs you may conceive?

Developing such a vision is the first step towards motivation. Motivation is the next step towards forming an idea or plan. A plan with proper discipline and execution leads to action. Constant action and activity leads to results. Results reinforce or enhance your vision of what you may become and inspires you to an even higher and more complete vision of total personal wellness. Nevertheless, it all starts with a specific vision that you are responsible to formulate and hold yourself accountable for. It begins with the vision of you seeing yourself at your best. That is a vision that anyone and everyone can aspire to.

A simple illustration of this visionary process is shown below:

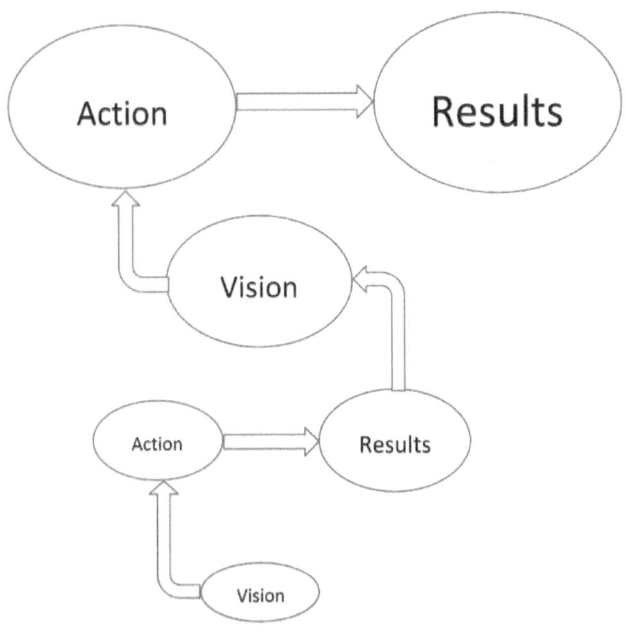

Vison-action-Results Diagram

The more you create a realistic vision that translates into sustainable actions, the more results you will see. The harvested results reinforce and expand that vision, confirming your developing philosophies and encouraging you to continue to grow that vision which leads to greater action and greater results. In wellness, as in many human endeavors, this model demonstrates the fundamental progress that is available to everyone, if we will simply choose to embark on that specific course. And what better or more satisfying vision than your own vision of complete wellness?

<u>Formulating a Plan</u>

Achieving personal wellness is not a random event. It does not happen by just thinking about it. Envisioning and dreaming of fitness of body and wellness of mind are no more than pleasant thoughts until you are seriously motivated to quantify what you want to do and how to do it. You can envision strong, defined muscles and endurance that would enable you to run for hours on end, but if you are not actually engaged on a regular basis in activities that increase strength and endurance it is no more than a daydream.

You can envision growing intellectual curiosity and the acquisition of greater knowledge and more coherent wisdom, but if you are not reading, studying, participating in professional developmental activities and so forth, your mind may remain comparatively sedentary. Or worse, be filled with useless and counterproductive information.

If you are ever to cross the divide that separates the sedentary and acted upon self into the proactive, fit and well self you must have a plan that will enable you to execute your vision of fitness and health. And it must be continually emphasized that you alone are responsible to decide what that plan will look like and how specifically it will be executed.

A plan for fitness must have certain characteristics if it is to be successful. First, it must be attractive to you. It has to include activities that you would find enjoyment and satisfaction in. Second, it must fit in with the larger picture of your daily life. If you are a busy executive, long two-hour excursions in the middle of the afternoon might not fit into your daily schedule. A busy housewife and mother with small children might have to find ways to plan activities where she receives assistance with her daily family responsibilities.

Third, your plan must be realistic. You cannot expect to gain strength and muscle mass without regular and strenuous resistance training. You cannot expect to build endurance without regular intervals that raise your heart rate and engage your muscles for extended periods. You cannot become more informed and intellectually rounded on a specialized subject without making time to read, research and ponder the things you seek to learn.

A realistic plan would play to your physiological strengths based on your body type, time constraints and overall vision for yourself. It must also accommodate time and space for your intellectual and spiritual interests. There must be room in a busy day to find space to pursue the more refined and ethereal subjects.

Fourth, your plan has to allow time for rest and recovery. It is sometimes possible to exercise too much as it is not to exercise enough. This is particularly true as you age or achieve significant fitness levels and continue to push hard to train to even higher goals.

Fifth, plans need to flexible. Your interests, activities, results and general circumstances may change over time. Do not be afraid to let your wellness plan change over time as your needs or opportunities change.

Sixth, your plan should equally accommodate the needs of mind, body and spirit. Each area has impact and importance on you overall wellness. Neglect in one domain may be compensated for somewhat in another, but not completely. The truly well person is cognizant and comfortable in all three of these aspects of self.

This relationship is simply illustrated below:

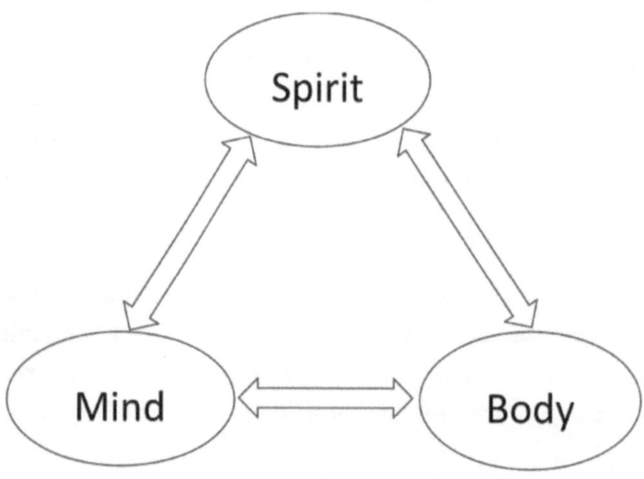

Body-Mind-Spirit Diagram

The combination of activities that strengthen these three aspects of self are the three cornerstones of a complete wellness philosophy. How you choose specifics in each of these three areas may be as unique as you are. There are generally no bad answers in wellness, just information that is more relevant or less relevant to where you want to be based on your own personal vision. The assumptions that advise your vision should be based on the most accurate information you can acquire.

The activities outlined in the subheadings below form a simplistic baseline for each area of consideration as you form, revise, or consistently evaluate your own wellness plan. As we will discuss further in Pathway #6, an appropriate balance in each of these areas is crucial to overall wellness.

Physical Fitness Plan; Wellness of Body

We will begin with the baseline physical activities that are associated with fitness based wellness. The minimum parameters for the three types of widely agreed upon physical activity, are discussed below. Your personal plan should take into consideration each of these physical parameters as you envision, analyze and execute a new or current exercise regimen or other physical activities.

Endurance Activities: Most experts agree that a minimum of three days per week with a minimum fifteen minutes per day of elevated cardiovascular activity is required to establish and maintain a baseline level of fitness. This means that whatever activity you engage in should elevate your heart and respiratory rate into a training zone of at least 65% of your maximum heart rate (based on age) for fifteen consecutive minutes at least three times per week. Most experts also agree that four to six days per week and longer intervals of twenty minutes to an hour or more will yield more rapid results and establish higher levels of cardiovascular fitness.

Some routines, such as training for marathons or triathlons, require several hours of training nearly every day of the week. Most experts agree that seven days per week is not necessary and there should be some down time for recuperation within a weekly routine. Achieving high levels of cardiovascular endurance definitely requires an investment in time. The greater the desired endurance, the more significant the investment of time required. Adequate time for maintaining flexibility and recovery should also be factored in when participating in higher level cardiovascular activities.

Strength Activities: Resistance training activities also require an investment of time. That time will also be somewhat proportional to your desired level of results. Resistance training activities can be achieved in smaller windows of time generally due to the short and intense nature of the exercises that increase strength. Most experts agree that a strength training routine should stimulate the desired muscle groups being trained at least two times and usually no more than three times per week.

Because of the recovery required from vigorous strength training, most fitness professionals would recommend a period of at least forty-two hours between working specific muscle groups. This is the minimum time required to rest and chemically recharge muscles to enable them to perform at peak efficiency for the next training session. Resistance training can be shortened into brief windows of thirty minutes of intense activity with little rest time, or extended into hour plus sessions of methodical and varied training routines.

Flexibility Activities: There is a very broad ongoing discussion regarding which types of flexibility exercises and how much stretching is required to maintain adequate levels of fitness. Some schools of thought prescribe equal time for stretching proportional to the time spent exercising. Other experts outline more, some outline much less.

Common sense should play a role in all of your fitness planning, but particularly when it comes to flexibility. Flexibility activities should be integrated into independent routines such as yoga and into pre-and post-workout routines with regularity. These should be done in an amount that feels effective and comfortable to you. Some physiological types, such as Ectomorphs, are naturally flexible and require less time and attention to maintain flexibility. Other types, such as Mesomorphs, may require extended stretching exercises to avoid losing muscular flexibility.

Some examples of fairly basic weekly exercise plans based on area of emphasis are illustrated below. Your personal exercise plan can be as creative and diverse as you wish to make it. Keep in mind there are numerous ways to exercise and no particular type of exercise is arguably the best, unless you decide it is. Your best plan is a plan that both encompasses the principles of the Twelve Pathways and keeps you engaged in the activities on a regular and consistent basis.

Examples of Area of Emphasis Exercise Plans:

Cardiovascular Oriented Fitness Plan – Monday: Walk minimum 30 minutes. Tuesday: Run 4 miles medium pace, stretch. Wednesday: bicycle for 45 minutes minimum, stretch. Thursday: Flex day – rest, stretch, yoga or hike for 30 minutes. Friday: Run for minimum 45 minutes, stretch. Saturday: Run 30 minutes and hike 30 Minutes. Sunday: Rest.

Strength Oriented Fitness Plan – Monday: Lift back and shoulders one hour, stretch. Tuesday: Lift chest one hour, stationary bike 20 minutes. Wednesday: Lift legs one hour, stretch. Thursday: Lift back and shoulders one hour. Friday: Lift chest one hour, stationary bike 30 minutes, stretch. Saturday: Lift legs 30 minutes, stationary bike. Sunday: Rest.

General Balanced Fitness Plan – Monday: Run for 45 minutes, stretch. Tuesday: Lift circuit training for upper body. Wednesday: Elliptical runner 30 minutes, lift circuit training for lower body, stretch. Thursday: Flex day, rest, yoga, stretch, walk. Friday: Lift upper body, stationary bike 20 minutes. Saturday: Run for 60 minutes, stretch. Sunday: Cross-fit training.

Examples of more specific plans and routines will be discussed in Pathway #7.

Whatever plans you adopt over time, determine to execute that plan faithfully. Goals can only be achieved and positive results realized if you regularly and consistently execute a fitness plan. Following a plan regularly requires discipline, but it also engenders discipline. You do not need to be perfect in executing a plan, but you need to remain steady and reliable in sticking to that plan. That discipline and steadiness begins with clear and realistic goals combined with a determination to fulfill them.

Keeping an Exercise Plan Record

If you have not established a specific exercise plan, start now by pondering what you want to accomplish and write down those goals and activities that are relevant to you. Keep a journal, use an app or track sheet on which you can write your goals down, then track your progress towards that goal. Just as an unwritten wish has a hard time becoming a goal, so an unwritten record of exercise results cannot become a direct indicator of your progress.

There are numerous exercise and nutrition oriented apps that can assist in identifying specific goals and activities. Applications such as RockMyRun, Edomondo, or MapMyFitness. These apps can receive manually uploaded workout data or be tied to personal fitness devices such as FitBit. Tracking sheets are useful when using resistance training exercises that cannot be tracked electronically. Journals may be more useful for tracking more fluid routines as well as recording feelings and impressions of a specific day's activities.

Whatever your goals and plan, keeping a consistent record of your accomplishments will allow you to clearly see progress. It also helps identify areas where you might be stagnating and need change or improvement in your routine. Keep a record and review that record periodically. It will reinforce the benefits and point out any weaknesses in your fitness plan.

Intellectual Plans; Strengthening the Mind

Just as the body requires regular activity, the mind also needs regular stimuli to remain healthy and sharp. Additionally, a broader acquisition of knowledge and wisdom leads to greater self-empowerment. It is only through a clear and accurate understanding of the world around you and the fundamental principles that define and govern that world that you can truly be empowered within the greater framework of complete wellness.

The beauty of stimulating the mind, and as a general definition we would use the idea of a continual education and storing of correct knowledge as the standard, is that our increase in mental acuity can continue to grow. One fact leads us to two more which leads us to four more and so on. One pearl of truth or wisdom sheds light on two more and so on. We can increase our "mental muscle" continually throughout our lives.

As sentient beings, we are capable of finding meaning wherever we choose to. This is both a gift and a responsibility. Every bit of knowledge we acquire we become responsible for. This is a natural process and should be seen as a joyful process within the context of complete wellness. How you should marvel at your own ability to increase in knowledge and wisdom!

But to increase in your intellectual abilities requires a commitment of time and relevant activities. A steady diet of Game Shows or Sitcoms does little to increase intellectual capabilities. However, the reading of a good book, fifteen minutes of a puzzle or word game, or studying a second language has been shown to increase brain activity and brain capacity.

Further, the human mind generally seeks stimulation. You are always thinking and becoming, each and every day, moment to moment. Your mind is always active, looking for something to fill the waking moments. You have to choose what you will fill your mind with. Complete wellness suggests that the things you "program" into your mind are going to be uplifting, informative and inspiring as well as stimulating.

Your mind is similar to your body in another way. If you feed it "mental junk food" you will quickly become intellectually unfit. The garbage in garbage out principle (discussed in detail in Pathway #8) applies every bit as much in intellectual pursuits. Wellness of mind implores you to remove the negative, cluttering "mental junk" and replace it with a healthy diet of information and ideas.

A simple example of this benefit is shown in a study by Nizam's Institute of Medical Sciences in Hyderabad, India. This study of 648 seniors found that those who studied and spoke a second language delayed the onset of Alzheimer's by nearly five years. A diet of useful information keeps the mind steady, active and engaged.

A basic intellectual plan should contain goals that reinforce wholesome mental activity. It might include such activities as:

Reading a new book every month
Joining a book club
Joining a bridge group
Writing a book on a subject of expertise
Writing an article each week for a local publication
Playing a stimulating online word game fifteen minutes per day
Studying a second language
Completing a crossword puzzle or Sudoku each day
Taking interesting continuing education classes

<u>Spiritual Wellness; Connecting with the Higher Self</u>

Spirituality is a very independent issue. Perceptions of spirituality are almost as unique as each individual. But there are significant commonalities that define our innate yearning for spiritual connection and meaning. Wellness of spirit, though interconnected with wellness of mind and body, has its own special considerations.

A personal spiritual journey often involves connecting with something larger than self. It seeks a broader and more metaphysical definition of meaning and purpose in life. In the context of wellness, the most important consideration is that you possess a sense of meaning and have avenues that can help translate that desire for meaning into tangible outlets that elevate you personally and others around you.

Productive spirituality often involves reaching outside of yourself and connecting with others and with the world around you in positive ways. This could be manifest in contemplative activities, where you seek enlightenment and deeper metaphysical understanding of the world and universe in which we live. Or it could involve more direct connection and activity by seeking opportunities to lift and serve others.

However you choose to pursue your own spiritual preferences, the point of the exercise is to nurture and grow this part of your being. Like your mind and body, you need to feed your spiritual self. For some this may come naturally, for others a distinct effort to grow this aspect may be necessary. It all depends on the combination of your natural spiritual inclinations and the cultural and societal expectations you have inherited.

Nurturing spiritual wellness should include regular activities that contribute to your perception of spiritual well-being. Such activities might include:

Volunteering at a Community Center once a month
Praying or meditating daily
Accepting a contributing role at a local church or other religious organization
Teaching a class on spiritual principles

Taking a humanitarian trip to serve an underprivileged community in another country

Reading or writing a spiritual ideas online blog

Attending regular religious services

Achieving Your Goals; Specifying Results

Wellness is a results oriented business. If you do not achieve what you set out to accomplish, sustaining any wellness lifestyle becomes more difficult. As mentioned previously, a wish that is not quantified as a goal is little more than a daydream. Any plan that you put together should have goals in mind. Your goals can be both general or more specific, simple or more complex, but should seek to quantify results.

You may have a goal to lose weight or reduce body fat. How can you translate that goal into results? How many pounds do you want to lose? How much body fat do you wish to burn? Will you take into account that as you train you may lose fat and gain muscle and that your actual weight might not change significantly in the long run?

Do you want to look better? Feel better? Be mentally sharper? Be more spiritually well-rounded? What does that specifically mean to you? These are all considerations that you should quantify by creating more simple and specific goals for yourself. Your goals need to be realistic and achievable. They should be based on expectations that you can meet with reasonable effort.

If you create more specific goals, it is easier to create a plan of action that targets those goals. You will be more effective at obtaining the results you initially envisioned and will therefore be more motivated to remain engaged in regular wellness activities. If you have already achieved significant wellness goals in a particular area, revisit those goals regularly. Make sure you are staying on a course that taking you to your envisioned result.

As you become more specific in setting your goals, also be specific in tracking your results. Tap into whatever wellness resources you have available and execute your plan to achieve the results your goals suggest. As you achieve specific results, periodically reevaluate and decide whether what you have accomplished is good enough or if there are higher accomplishments you feel inspired to reach. Then simply move forward and do it. Keep doing it. Make it happen and change yourself and your life forever.

Some examples of general and specific fitness oriented wellness goals you might consider are listed below. Note that each general goal has a specific example. There may be many specific goals associated with the accomplishment of an overarching general goal:

General Goals	Specific Goals
Lose Weight	Lose X pounds by Y date
Build endurance	Be able to run 2 miles in fifteen minutes
Increase strength	Be able to do 30 push-ups per day
Increase muscle mass	Increase chest size from X to Y
Reduce body fat	Decrease waist size from X to Y in 3 months
Feel healthier	Be able to walk up 4 flights of stairs with ease
Look better	Reduce body fat X percent
Feel stronger	Be able to row for half an hour
Have more energy	Be able to walk for one hour
Have more clarity of thought	Read a book for one hour uninterrupted
Become more service oriented	Serve in a local homeless shelter 1x per month
Stretch spiritual boundaries	Take a humanitarian vacation to Africa
Increase mental capacity	Study Japanese or Chinese for 20 mins. per day
Increase scientific knowledge	Take a class in physiology online

<u>Quick Tips on Creating a Wellness Plan</u>

- Create a goal sheet. Establish general and specific goals. Tie those goals to your fitness journal.
- Record specific workout results and track your progress on an exercise log.
- Purchase a Fitbit or other activity tracker. Use the accompanying app to create data history.
- Join with a workout partner in supporting your mutual fitness goals. Establish goals and timelines and reward each other for your accomplishments.
- Create weekly or monthly mission statements. Display the new mission statement each week or month and honestly evaluate your achievements.
- Plan a community oriented activity. Invite family and friends.
- Create target events, such as a series of annual races in your community. Enter these events each time they are held and compare your season to season progress.
- Have an annual Body Composition Analysis and an annual physical and create a record book of your compositional and medical status.
- Create a reading list. Include at least four books you find stimulating.
- Establish a fitness journal. Include events, pictures, goals, times, achievements, exercise logs, diet logs and any other materials that are of interest and can help you track your progress.

OVERALL BALANCE IS CRITICAL, IN WELLNESS AND IN LIFE

Whatever plans and goals you make, a key principle to overall and ongoing wellness is balance. To be able to sustain a wellness lifestyle long term, you must have the concept of balance built into your daily routines and activities. You must work your body in ways that achieve balance in your conditioning. You must feed your mind and spirit with useful and uplifting information.

Keep in mind balance can mean different things to different people depending on their personal vision and goals. Nevertheless, there are a few basic and essential concepts of balance that are critical to incorporate into any plan to sustain overall wellness, maintaining body symmetry, mental clarity minimize the possibility of injury, illness or distress over time.

You need to achieve balanced both internally and externally. Internal balance involves critical organs such as the heart, lungs, digestive system and your circulatory system. It also involves a mental and spiritual balance that involved active and clear thought processes, reasoning and spiritual intuition. External balance involves your musculature and joints as they support your skeletal system.

Internal Physical and Intellectual Balance

Your internal systems are not visible when you look at yourself in a mirror. You cannot see the functions of organs such as your heart, liver, lungs and stomach. You cannot map your mind working even though your thoughts may be deep or poignant. But these systems are critical to your overall health. They experience wear and tear every bit the equivalent of the external and visible systems of your body.

In fact, it can be argued that as you get older, the most important systems in your body are your brain, heart and lungs. Circulatory health affects every other function of your body. Heart disease, diabetes, cancer, stroke and many other dangers to your health all have association with poor cardiovascular performance. Deterioration in brain function can rob you of a healthy and full lifestyle. If your heart is unhealthy, it may not matter how well other systems are functioning as heart problems can often be fatal.

Internal balance in your body comes from incorporating a minimum recommended amount of cardiovascular activity with proper nutrition and hydration. All the muscular strength in the world will be fruitless if it is not supported by healthy internal systems. Your body needs regular activity that raises your heart rate and forces your lungs and circulatory systems to work at elevated levels for sustained periods of time. The functional human body needs cardiovascular stimulation. It responds well to consistent levels of cardiovascular work. The stomach, liver and other organs will function more efficiently when your cardiovascular health is at peak performance. You remove waste more effectively from your body. You sleep more effectively and digest your food more thoroughly and efficiently. Mental functions are increased due to more efficient blood and oxygen flow throughout the brain.

Balance is also reflected in maintaining the proper ratios of muscle mass, body fat and bone density based on your physical body type. When you are well conditioned, your body naturally maintains a healthy balance in these three areas. Excessive body fat as a percentage of overall body weight is an indicator of numerous internal ailments including diabetes, heart disease and stroke. Lack of muscle mass in relation to overall body weight slows the overall metabolism compared to more balanced muscle weight densities.

Healthy body fat levels, healthy muscle mass, bone density and healthy marrow counts are directly linked to properly functioning immunity levels. The advantages of maintaining cardiovascular and muscular health are key to the balanced functioning of all of these related internal systems. Consistent activity based wellness not only helps you look better on the outside, but helps you function better internally as well.

Balance of the mind is linked inextricably with physical conditions. Under normal physical conditions the brain is receiving proper nutrients and hydration. Proper nutrition helps the brain maintain balanced and healthy neurological functions. With healthy blood flow, the brain is well oxygenated and your focus and mental acuity remains sharper longer.

There are numerous ways to "feed the brain" nutritionally that contribute to healthy brain function. Foods such as raisins, blueberries and avocados have been shown to support healthy brain activity. Foods with high levels of sugar or diet soda have been shown to actually impair mental function.

You cannot externally measure healthy cognitive function. A healthy mind contributes to a healthy attitude. A healthy physical attitude encourages proper activities. Proper activities are manifest in your external appearance and function. Further, healthy cognitive function is apparent in your speech and mannerisms.

External Physical Balance

Your physical activities should take into account the fact that your body's musculature functions in specific ways. Muscles move through specific ranges of motion. The body consists of diametrically opposed muscle groups that support the skeletal system through various movements. You should always incorporate concepts of balance that properly and equally train opposing muscle groups to maintain overall strength balance throughout your body. You should also incorporate a balance of strength and endurance activities for various muscle groups depending upon your overall fitness goals.

When training for either strength or endurance it is important to consider the balancing functions of opposing muscle groups. There are certain parts of the musculoskeletal system that push or pull in opposing motions. It is important for overall health that these muscles are conditioned equally and work in balance one against the other. The key to balance is that if you work one group of muscles you must give equal and adequate work to the other opposing group. The major opposing muscle group areas include:

<u>"Pushing" Muscles</u>	<u>Opposing "Pulling" Muscles</u>
Triceps	(arms) Biceps (arms)
Pectorals (chest)	Latissimus Dorsi (back)
Abdominals (stomach)	Erector Spinae (lower back)
Quadriceps (legs)	Hamstrings (legs)
Adductors (legs)	Abductors (legs)

Lack of balance between opposing muscle groups over time will lead to strength imbalances that can compromise the appearance and symmetry of your body as well increase the likelihood of injury to the imbalanced areas. For example, a very strong chest without equally conditioned back muscles can pull the entire shoulder girdle forward, pulling the upper back, head and neck out of alignment. This compromises posture and opens the area up for discomfort or injury to the back and neck.

External balance is further demonstrated in combining a strong musculature structure with a strong cardiovascular system. Unless you are training for specific competitive activities such as bodybuilding, team sports or running marathons, the best overall fitness plans incorporate both strength and endurance. It is equally important to have strong muscles and healthy joints as it is to have endurance and a healthy cardiovascular system. Balance between the two ideals of size and strength versus stamina should be considered in any fitness plan.

Balancing Large to Small Muscle Groups

A significant part of exercise theory involves working from large to small muscle groups. When you are formulating more specific exercise routines, not just general wellness activities that involve overall movement, it is important to work your body in sequences that take advantage of your muscular ability to reach a point of beneficial hypertrophy. This applies most specifically to resistance oriented training, where your highest benefits are achieved when you work muscles to the point of momentary failure.

It is critical that your activities move from large muscle group movements that engage numerous interconnected muscles simultaneously, down to more isolated and specific muscles. For example, if strengthening your lower body, including legs and gluteus muscles, is your goal then a large body movement would include squats or lunges. A more isolated body movement would include leg extension, leg curl or calf raise.

The large body movements engage most of the leg muscles at once. The isolated movements engage only the muscle groups targeted, such as the calves or hamstrings. Most fitness routines oriented towards general fitness (not a sport specific routine) recommend a mixture of both large muscle movements combined with specific isolated muscle movements. Modern research generally agrees that if strength increases are a goal then performing regular large movements are critical in increasing overall body strength.

It is important to engage large muscles movements first before moving on to more specific muscles unless you are designing a specific pre-exhaust/post exhaust routine. For example, if your goal is to exercise your back, you will need to engage your arms and biceps in movements involving your back muscles. If you have previously done isolated exercise for your biceps, they will be too exhausted to effectively work your back muscles. Your arms will give out before your back has reached a level of effective training.

Working from large to small is important in resistance oriented activities. The same applies in cross training situations. You do not want to work smaller more isolated areas of your body if they are going to be needed shortly for large movements. Again, the exception would be a pre-exhaust/ post exhaust routine for specific isolated muscles. For example, in isolating biceps, arm curls may be followed by negative only pullups using connecting muscles to super exhaust the smaller group.

Balance of Mind and Spirit

If wellness is to become a way of life, by implication your outlook and activity must encompass more than the physical. Many types of activities, particularly eastern disciplines such as Tae Kwon Do, Tai Chi and Yoga, blend mental and spiritual focus with physical exertion. A physically sound body supports a fitter mind and deeper spiritual commitment, and vice versa.

If you are disciplined enough to maintain a daily fitness routine, you have likely also developed a portion of your character that engenders respect, commitment and care. Your overall levels of wellness are more balanced if your entire focus is on more than just the physical. As illustrated in Pathway #5, exercising your mind, stimulating your intellect and developing a curiosity for things cerebral and metaphysical have been shown to reinforce a positive view of self.

Spiritual balance is more easily achieved when you can internalize a perspective of the importance of the metaphysical within the context of the everyday world. Spiritual meaning is interpreted very personally and individually, but can play a critical role in defining your own self-concept. We all establish our own spiritual priorities, whether they are based on culture, religion or other definitive frameworks.

Overall wellness suggests that you nurture those spiritual needs equally with physical needs. There is a lot of research associating wellness of mind and spirit with wellness of body. In other words, even though we cannot see the results of spiritual well-being in a mirror, our spiritual and mental states may have a direct effect on the vibrancy of physical health. A happy mind assists in a healthy body and vice versa.

Balance applies to the mind and spirit as you spend the time and effort necessary to develop these less tangible, but equally important, aspects of self. Your life will be fuller, richer and more gratifying if you nurture all three aspects of your being. Mind, body and spirit are inescapably intertwined. Health in one area supports health in another. Lack of health in one requires compensation from another or imbalance may result.

Intellectual pursuits such as reading, arts and crafts, community service or hobbies contribute to a fuller balance of self. So do spiritual pursuits of worship, prayer, humanitarian work or meditation. Whatever your interest, pursue them well and with enthusiasm. Become well-rounded in each aspect of self. You and all those with whom you work and live will become the ultimate beneficiaries.

Quick Tips for Achieving Overall Balance

- In a workout diary, document the number of routines that involve opposing body parts, see if opposing numbers remain roughly equal from month to month.
- Stagger your routines. Switch between strength and cardio routines on alternating weeks. Use a 4-2, 2-4, 4-2, 2-4 pattern over the course of a month instead of 3-3 predictable schedule.
- If you are challenged with strength training, try integrating high intensity push-pull routines, such as rapid station circuit training, into a weekly routine.
- If you are challenged with cardio balance, integrate 15-20 minutes of stationary biking or elliptical training as a warm up for strength routines.

- Meet with a training professional at least once a month to evaluate and obtain a second opinion on your exercise schedules and routines.
- Try to integrate at least fifteen minutes of stretching for every hour of your exercise routine.
- Take a martial arts class and learn both the principles and the movements.
- Try yoga or meditation at least every other week for a change of pace.
- Join a local community service organization; look for meaningful projects to enrich others.
- Start a book club with friends and challenge each other to read stimulating material.
- Take at least ten to fifteen minutes per day for meditation or prayer.
- Relax, take a weekend vacation, play a word game online, watch the sunset.
- Write a monthly special interest article for a local newspaper.

VARIETY IS THE SPICE OF LIFE AND A KEY TO WELLNESS ALSO

Now is a great time to be engaged in personal wellness. Decades of research have yielded new and exciting ways to exercise and develop the body and mind. Techniques and insights that were unheard of thirty years ago are matter-of-fact today. There seems to be no end to the activities, programs and ideas dedicated to wellness concepts. Employers have discovered the benefits of wellness and the value wellness brings to individual employees. Programs, challenges, online applications and other tools are numerous. Technologies supporting wellness oriented activities continue to be developed and improve constantly. As with most developments in fields of this type, information and understanding tends to increase exponentially over time.

This is very beneficial if you are an aspiring or established fitness enthusiast. One of the more advanced but often overlooked principles of wellness is to understand that your body and mind actually crave a variety of activities. The more numerous and varied activities you can engage in and master, the better results you will see in the long run. The average person naturally trends toward that which is familiar and comfortable. Change is frequently seen as a stressor. Wellness suggests change and variety should be embraced as an opportunity. And there has never been a greater abundance and variety of activities available than there are today.

The human body likes a mixture of different physical stimuli. While the best form of activity is the one you will stick with most diligently, a variety of activities will be more effective in the long run. One type of activity can provide a foundation to be successful at other pursuits. Different activities can synergize and build upon one another. Not only will variety in the types and programs of activities you engage in keep you mentally fresh and excited about exploring new or different avenues of wellness, it will bring greater results over time if you mix things up.

The mind is likewise receptive to varied activity. To spend excessive amounts of time on one mental pursuit can lead to burn out. Changing up your inspirations, studying different subjects, perhaps some light, some heavy, some just entertaining, keeps your intellect engaged. We now live in a world of nearly unlimited information. Choose a variety of subjects to enhance your curiosity and learning, and choose them well.

Two Barriers to Complete Wellness

There are two major barriers that will inhibit your ability to establish and execute an ongoing and sustainable wellness plan. The first barrier is the "entry barrier." This barrier consists of negative thoughts or behavioral patterns that inhibit you from choosing to engage in daily activity that will improve your wellness. These patterns can arise for a number of reasons. It may be the erroneous idea that exercise or other activities are too difficult or too time consuming. It might revolve around a general misunderstanding of exactly how to get started. It may just be attributable to a lack of social support or encouragement from those in positions of trust.

If you have led a sedentary lifestyle for an extended time, this entry barrier can also be manifest in the physical strain and discomfort of beginning an exercise program. When your body is not used to activity, it takes some time to "get over the hump" when starting consistent and strenuous movement. This initial physical entry barrier can last from several weeks to many months depending on your current physical condition.

You should always begin a new series of activities slowly and gradually. It is recommended that if you have been sedentary for a number of years that you undergo a physical and incorporate any medical restrictions or cautions into your program. But the whole idea behind wellness is to start moving, then keep moving, increasing your activities as you are physically able. Whatever the reasons, mental or physical, any entry barrier must be addressed and overcome before positive daily habits can be integrated into a beneficial wellness lifestyle.

The second barrier is known as the "progress barrier." A common term for this barrier in fitness parlance is known as "hitting a plateau." This occurs when established habits, practices or routines become so repetitive that the body stops responding to a specific stimulus at an ascending rate. As a general rule, your body needs to be stimulated to a certain level for the physiological changes necessary for increased fitness to occur. When a stimulus is adapted to by the body, the physiological changes decrease or cease altogether. It is at this point that progress flattens, or a "plateau" occurs.

The mind is also similar. Receiving the same information day in and day out sets mental processes on "automatic". You may be receiving information and using as little mental exertion as possible to process that data. Your mind gets stale, and you do not use even a fraction of your intellectual capacity in such routine. It requires a change, a challenge, a fun diversion of thought or contemplation to keep the mind operating on a high level.

Physical exertion, when looked at from a purely physiological perspective, is simply your body's adaptation to stresses being put upon it. The body's reactions to the stresses of exercise result in increased strength, muscle mass and cardiovascular efficiency. You must engage in aerobic activity for a sustained period several times a week to consistently stress the body's cardiovascular system. For strength training, muscles need to be stimulated to levels of momentary failure consistently for growth to occur.

However, if the same exercises are used to achieve these results again and again, over a period of weeks or months, the body adapts and becomes used to these stimuli. The body compensates for specific exercise stimuli and learns to dull the response to these stimuli. Gains slow or become stagnant. Cardiovascular performance reaches a level and stays at that level or even declines.

When a plateau is reached it is often the first inclination to do more of the same activities, only harder, heavier, more frequently and more intensely than before to try and break through and increase results. This is a natural reaction to a lack of response to established routine. Pushing harder versus changing the nature of the routine is often a precursor to injury or exhaustion. Adding variety to your activities is the best solution to continually escalating or maintaining specific physical goals and targets. If your progress hits a plateau, simply try something new or different.

You may hit a plateau for many reasons. Perhaps you have not understood the benefits of variety and have not envisioned a diverse routine. Perhaps you have become very comfortable with your training routines and like to keep things conveniently within the scope of your favorite activities. Perhaps you have been pushing so hard on a given routine you're your body is actually over trained and needs rest, change and recovery. Perhaps a lack of time or unclear results have prevented incorporating more variety.

Whatever the reasons a plateau may occur, resolve to be creative and explore new and interesting activities. Who knows what fun you may be missing? Envision new and exciting horizons ahead, with even greater results than you might have imagined.

Change Your Routines Periodically

When it comes to physical variety, it is more natural to trend toward those activities we are most comfortable with. We tend to stick with what has worked in the past. Routines and programs can become too repetitive and thus progress slows. There are many modern types of activity that seek to incorporate concepts of "muscle confusion" or cross-fit training principles. These types of activities have been designed to address many of the issues that training plateaus produce. They incorporate a differing variety of movements into a given routine. Then they change the routine itself on a regular basis.

Research has shown that the body responds more quickly to stimulation that stresses the body in different and unpredictable ways. The principle is fairly simple. You should consider rotating the activities you do regularly to allow your body to react to new and different stimuli while avoiding long periods of time at repetitive activities. Mentally, it can be refreshing to get out of your "comfort zone" from time to time. The anticipation of trying something new can often be more stimulating than intimidating.

This can be accomplished by having a series of exercises that you do for a few weeks at a time for each series. It can also be accomplished by alternating movements within a given routine. Most modern training experts would agree with the idea that you should never continue to do one specific type or routine of exercise for lengthy extended periods. Given enough time and enough adaptation by the body, hitting a sustained plateau and halting your progress becomes counterproductive and may lead to loss of interest altogether.

As with any exercise program, the variety of activities and new exercises that may be incorporated are an open book. There are many options. Can you envision new and creative ways to keep moving that are personally exciting and appealing? One way to achieve this is to talk with other fitness friends or read a variety of literature with new ideas. Online resources and programs are plentiful. There are numerous ways to incorporate variety into daily activities, regardless of your available time frame.

It may be as simple as picking up a new piece of equipment to incorporate into a new routine. Perhaps running is a little stale and a bicycle or rowing machine would make a nice change-up. Perhaps a new variety of aerobics or fitness dancing has an appeal you may not have considered previously. Whatever your mind set, remember that variety is a good thing. It is a positive to have a regular routine that you will stick with and gets you out of bed in the morning. It is even better to have those regular activities change from time to time to keep things fresh and exciting and to keep moving in a productive direction that consistently yields results.

For purposes of illustration, examples of routine variation is illustrated below. Each routine is outlined to be sustained for a two to six week period. Rotation through several months of alternating A, B, C, D, E and F routines would encompass a thorough cross-fit philosophy. The routines are geared toward general balanced fitness approach for an individual with an intermediate level of fitness. Even the mix of exercises in the overall daily regimen could be varied in future iterations of the routines:

Routine A:

Monday	Tuesday	Wednesday	Thursday	Friday	Saturday
Run 30 min.	Lift Legs	Lift upper body	Run 40 min.	Cross-fit	Aerobics

Routine B:

Monday	Tuesday	Wednesday	Thursday	Friday	Saturday
Cross-fit	Bike 45 min.	Circuit Training	Yoga	Run 40 min.	Circuit Train

Routine C:

Monday	Tuesday	Wednesday	Thursday	Friday	Saturday
Zumba	Power Pump	Cycling	RIPPED	Yoga	Pilates

Routine D:

Monday	Tuesday	Wednesday	Thursday	Friday	Saturday
Rock Climbing	Speed Training	Strength training	Endurance run	Swimming	Walk & stretch

Routine E:

Monday	Tuesday	Wednesday	Thursday	Friday	Saturday
Rowing 1 hr.	Lift Up. Body	Plyometrics	Bike 1 hr.	Circuit Train	Walking 1 hr.

Routine F:

Monday	Tuesday	Wednesday	Thursday	Friday	Saturday
Boot camp	Racquetball	Hiking	Racquetball	Circuit training	Boxing

In summary, when it comes to wellness, variety is indeed a pleasant flavor for a complete wellness program. If you are keeping records of fitness goals and progress as outlined in Pathway #5, it becomes very easy to spot plateaus in your routine. Seek to negate these plateaus by incorporating variations into your exercise regimen. By doing so, you will keep your progress moving forward and perhaps explore new and interesting ways to incorporate fitness activities into your lifestyle.

Quick Tips for Maintaining Variety

- Take advantage of seasonal opportunities such as cross country skiing, downhill skiing, mountain biking, wilderness hiking, road races, mountain climbing, kayaking, canoeing, swimming, golf or other outdoor sports.
- Take a personal training course at a local career college and learn new training techniques.

- Look for fitness clubs in your community that support a wide variety of activities.
- Book several sessions with a reputable personal trainer and brainstorm new exercises that would appeal to you.
- Create a "bucket list" of fitness goals you would like to achieve, e.g. "Hike the glacier to the top of Mount Rainier, Washington" or "complete a full triathlon within one year."
- Keep a fitness journal, review your activities over the past six months. Make a plan to change any routine that has predominated more than 50% of your exercise time.
- Create a neighborhood fitness group that meets one day per week and assign each member as an activity leader for their respective week.
- If you are engaged in weight or circuit training, learn negative only, pre-exhaust – post – exhaust and drop-set routines to give additional variances to your established movements.
- Buy and read a book outside of your normal scope of interest. Share your new insights with a friend.
- Create a "healthy restaurant of the month club". Explore new places that offer healthy cuisine.
- Take a course that teaches a new computer skill you can apply in your professional life.

GARBAGE IN GARBAGE OUT; YOU MUST PROPERLY FEED AND HYDRATE YOUR MACHINE.

The human body is a marvel of complex biological engineering. It can be viewed as a wonderful and masterfully functioning system, a programmable biological machine. It responds to a wide variety of inputs, can create an incredible catalog of outputs and is able to heal and repair itself and keep on functioning through a remarkable range of conditions, favorable or difficult. Centuries of experience and the painstaking research of modern science continue to explore and reveal the mysterious and marvelous mechanism that comprise the human body. And we have only scratched the surface of discovery with regard to this amazing mechanism.

How many of the autonomous functions of the human body operate sustainably is still under investigation. We have much yet to discover. Through this entire history of discovery, one universally true principle has been confirmed time and again. What you use to feed and fuel your body will have a direct effect on how well your body develops and functions. If you put good nutrition in, you will generally get good health out. If you put poor nutrition in, the body will eventually break down and become unwell.

Nutrition is a very broad and complicated discipline. Orthodoxy surrounding optimal nutrition seems to be ever evolving and changing. Old paradigms of protein and carbohydrate based nutritional models are giving way to more plant based models. Regardless of the model or specific programs, it is evident that nutrition directly and profoundly effects the functioning of your body. Your weight, energy levels, stamina, blood sugar levels and even your mental functions have been linked in one way or another to the types of food you eat. "You are what you eat" is essentially fact. Your daily dietary choices will have a direct impact on your long term health.

Development of USDA Recommended Nutrition Standards

The United States Department of Agriculture (USDA) has incorporated the latest ideas in nutritional research into published standards. These standards have been around since 1916 and serve as a solid starting point to develop a nutrition plan. As nutritional research has progressed and new data is gathered, standards have been modified over time.

The basic modern standard for nutrition began with the Food Pyramid, originally published in 1992. This standard progressed into the MyPyramid in 2005 and the Food Plate in 2011. This framework seeks to establish a baseline for a normal "healthy" dietary standards. Wellness research tends to support the basic ideas of the Food Plate, but disagreement on what constitutes "real" food or the most ideal food options in the various categories is an ongoing discussion.

The food categories and proportions of various category types that constitute a healthy mixture of nutrition as outlined in the Food Plate are generally agreed upon by most wellness and nutrition experts. However, this does not mean that these recommendations are hard and fast nutritional truths. They are general guidelines.

The Food Plate outlines the basic food groups including breads and grains, fruits and vegetables, meats and proteins, and dairy. It illustrates them in a roughly proportional visual model, leaving specifics to exact amounts and types of each food group up to the individual. The past pyramid models were more specific in their recommendations.

Your body type, physical routines and personal preferences will also determine the proper diet for you to maintain high levels of personal wellness. The past two Food Pyramids and the current Food Plate outlining recommended daily servings of various food groups are illustrated below:

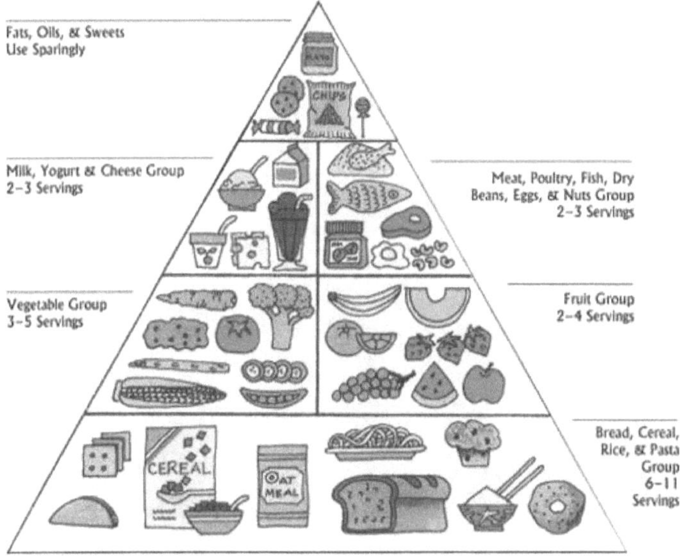

Original USDA Food Pyramid 1992

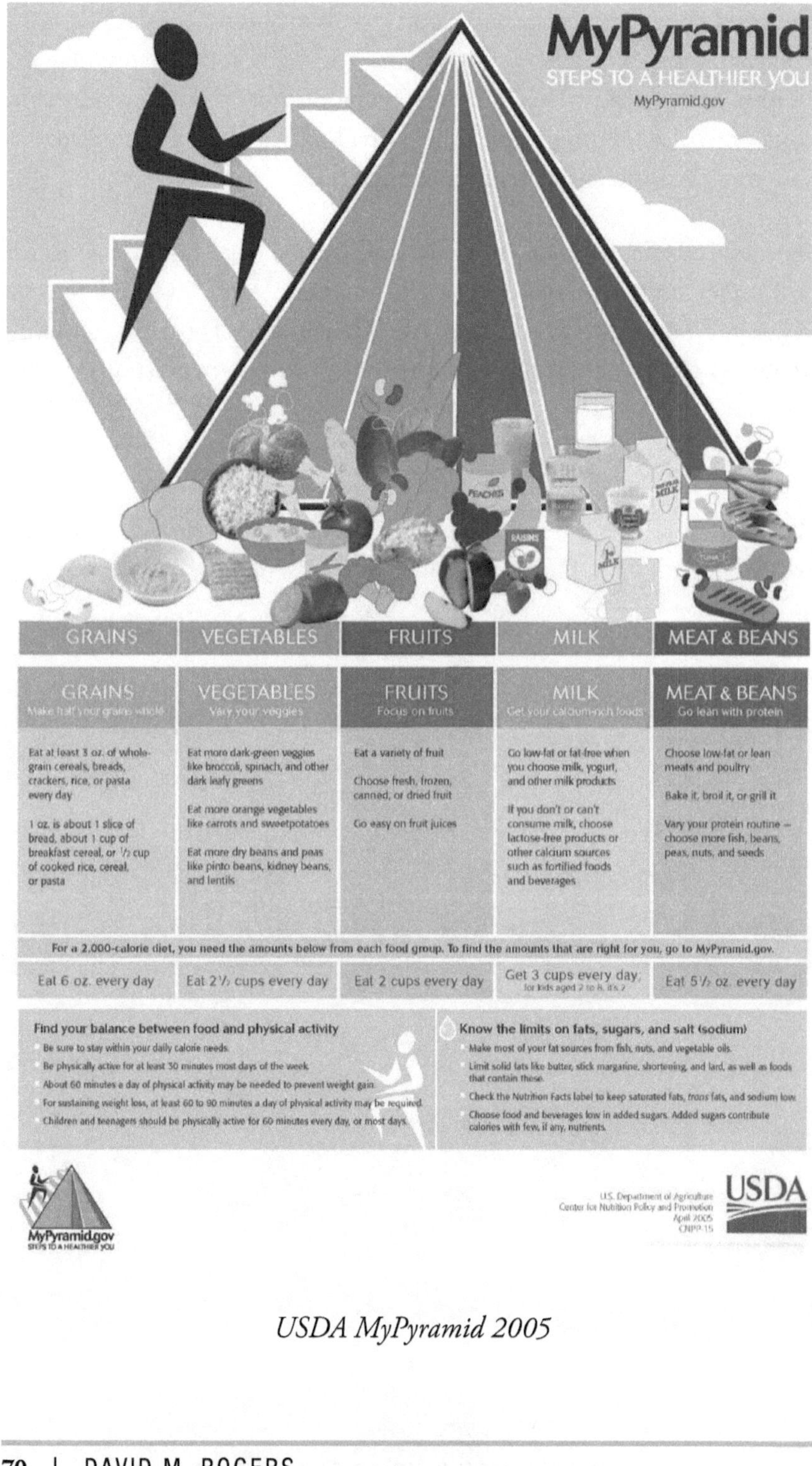

MyPyramid

STEPS TO A HEALTHIER YOU

MyPyramid.gov

GRAINS	VEGETABLES	FRUITS	MILK	MEAT & BEANS
GRAINS Make half your grains whole	**VEGETABLES** Vary your veggies	**FRUITS** Focus on fruits	**MILK** Get your calcium-rich foods	**MEAT & BEANS** Go lean with protein
Eat at least 3 oz. of whole-grain cereals, breads, crackers, rice, or pasta every day 1 oz. is about 1 slice of bread, about 1 cup of breakfast cereal, or ½ cup of cooked rice, cereal, or pasta	Eat more dark-green veggies like broccoli, spinach, and other dark leafy greens Eat more orange vegetables like carrots and sweetpotatoes Eat more dry beans and peas like pinto beans, kidney beans, and lentils	Eat a variety of fruit Choose fresh, frozen, canned, or dried fruit Go easy on fruit juices	Go low-fat or fat-free when you choose milk, yogurt, and other milk products If you don't or can't consume milk, choose lactose-free products or other calcium sources such as fortified foods and beverages	Choose low-fat or lean meats and poultry Bake it, broil it, or grill it Vary your protein routine — choose more fish, beans, peas, nuts, and seeds

For a 2,000-calorie diet, you need the amounts below from each food group. To find the amounts that are right for you, go to MyPyramid.gov.

Eat 6 oz. every day	Eat 2½ cups every day	Eat 2 cups every day	Get 3 cups every day. for kids aged 2 to 8, it's 2	Eat 5½ oz. every day

Find your balance between food and physical activity

- Be sure to stay within your daily calorie needs.
- Be physically active for at least 30 minutes most days of the week.
- About 60 minutes a day of physical activity may be needed to prevent weight gain.
- For sustaining weight loss, at least 60 to 90 minutes a day of physical activity may be required.
- Children and teenagers should be physically active for 60 minutes every day, or most days.

Know the limits on fats, sugars, and salt (sodium)

- Make most of your fat sources from fish, nuts, and vegetable oils.
- Limit solid fats like butter, stick margarine, shortening, and lard, as well as foods that contain these.
- Check the Nutrition Facts label to keep saturated fats, trans fats, and sodium low.
- Choose food and beverages low in added sugars. Added sugars contribute calories with few, if any, nutrients.

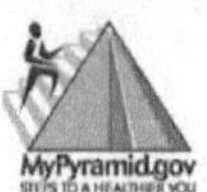

U.S. Department of Agriculture
Center for Nutrition Policy and Promotion
April 2005
CNPP-15

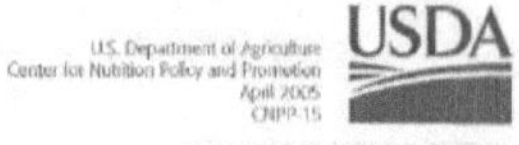

USDA MyPyramid 2005

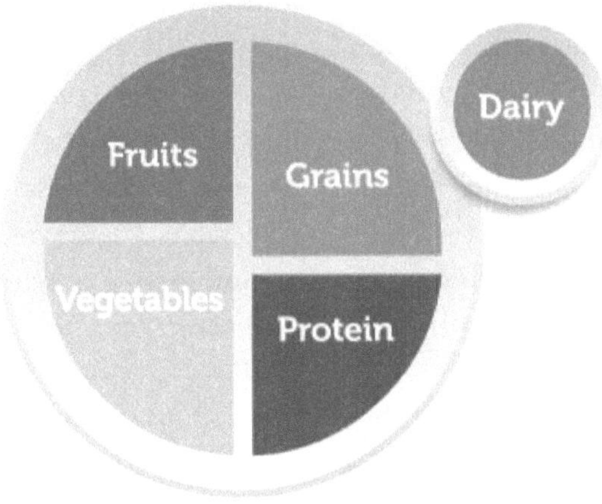

USDA Food Plate 2011

Eat a Variety of Foods

We all have our favorite foods–things that delight our taste buds and sate our appetites. Many of our eating habits are established at young ages, being passed down from parent to child. Many food preferences can be attributed to cultural upbringing and the concepts of "proper foods" that have been passed down through generations. These inbred ideas of what constitutes a meal can be uplifting, comforting and confirming in the identity of self or community. There is great psychological power and comfort latent in the concepts of how and what we feed ourselves.

However, within the context of achieving high levels of personal wellness, many of the concepts of food that you might have inherited over the years may be counterproductive to a healthy weight and wellness lifestyle. The great American tradition of hamburgers and hot dogs is just one of a multitude of examples where the food with which one is most familiar and induces the greatest culinary comfort and recognition might be the least healthy choice.

We live in an era where the variety of ideas and concepts of a healthy diet are as numerous as the people who propose them. The number of foods available today is staggering and can be almost confusing. Among all of this, simple principles exist to guide you in the choice of what might constitute the best diet for your lifestyle and wellness needs. The first guideline is that a variety of foods is preferable. A wide variety in your diet will more likely provide you with the combination of nutrients needed to fuel your body to its highest levels of performance.

The main areas of nutrition that any diet should address are the amounts of protein, carbohydrates, fats, fiber and vitamins and minerals the diet provides. Proteins are obtained through foods that contain a complete inventory of essential amino acids that rebuild muscle tissue and renew the body at a cellular level. Such foods include meat, fish, dairy products, nuts, seeds and legumes. Vegetarian diets seek to establish combinations of protein rich plant based foods and legumes to obtain all of the necessary proteins to keep the body renewed and healthy.

Carbohydrates consist of two varieties, simple and complex. Simple carbohydrates are obtained through foods rich in sugars, either artificial or natural. Simple carbohydrates are found in processed foods such as cookies or cake, and in natural foods such as oranges or pomegranates. Simple carbohydrates provide quick, short term energy. Complex carbohydrates are found mainly in grains such as wheat, rice, oats and barley. Complex carbohydrates must be broken down into simple carbohydrates within the body after they are eaten and therefore provide longer term energy.

Vitamins and minerals are also crucial to overall health. While some vitamins are found in foods that provide protein and carbohydrates, the densest source of vitamins and minerals is usually found in anti-oxidant rich fruits and vegetables. Fiber is found abundantly in almost any plant based vegetable or grain as well as in nuts and seeds.

Plant based diets are increasingly shown to be the most healthy for a wide variety of people. The natural vitamins and fiber, phytonutrients and lack of harmful fats that a primarily plant based diet contains have been shown to promote numerous health benefits. Modern diets tend to be far too carbohydrate rich. Excess carbohydrates are immediately stored as fat if they are not burned off through daily activity. Plant based diets provide easier-to-use calories and avoid fat buildup that result from carbohydrate heavy diets.

With the variety of nutrients needed for the body to maintain health, it would be wise to incorporate the types of food that will provide these diverse and necessary nutrients. This takes some thought and planning. Ratios of proteins to carbohydrates and the best sources of phytonutrients, vitamins and minerals vary from person to person and from body type to body type. Although it takes some work, a diet consisting of a balanced mixture of each of these foods will ultimately sustain health and reinforce the body and mind over time.

It is no coincidence that experts in wellness take great interest and spend significant time researching and planning wholesome and varied menus. Not only does this encourage the trying of new foods, new tastes and new possibilities, it allows your body to more effectively absorb the many needed nutritional requirements to remain in peak condition.

You Must Eat to be Fit

One of the great myths perpetuated over the years posits that low calorie "crash" diets are an effective path to weight loss and better health. This is actually the opposite of the facts established by research into diet and performance. Your body requires a certain baseline of calories each day to remain healthy. If you do not consume enough calories in the proper balance, you can actually do your body more harm than good.

If you reduce your caloric intake below what your body needs to maintain its basic functions, your body will react by going into "starvation mode". This means your metabolic rate will start to drop and your body will try to store as much fat as possible to prepare against further caloric deficits. Further, after you have resumed a more normal caloric intake, your body may store fat and gain weight even faster than prior to your diet.

The truth is that regular quality calorie intake is necessary to maintain proper weight and physical performance. The key focus centers on what specific foods you eat and how much of them you eat. Another key involves how often you eat. Research supports the idea that several smaller meals throughout the day keep your metabolic rate high. By eating smaller portions of healthy food more often you "keep your metabolic furnace stoked." This is obviously different than the traditional model of larger "breakfast, lunch, dinner" dining schedules many of us are accustomed to.

If you are used to consuming more calories than your body can use on a daily basis, reducing caloric input to a point where your body can restore metabolic balance and reduce fat levels is advisable. But this is a balancing act that you must consider carefully. Diets that severely reduce caloric intake are not a positive solution to better wellness, and often lead to more problems than benefits.

Proper Portions Equal Ideal Energy and Weight

As important as it is to incorporate a variety of foods to ensure adequate nutrition, it is equally important to eat the appropriate amounts of food given your body type and activity levels. The rule is simple: if you ingest more calories than you are able to burn in a day through activity and your natural metabolism, you will store the excess calories as fat. It does not matter what type or variety of calories are consumed, excess calories are not beneficial to overall wellness levels.

The portions of different food types consumed are equally significant. Variety in your diet helps you avoid consuming to much of one type of nutrient or another. Diets high in protein and animal fat can be problematic and create health problems. Diets rich in fruits and vegetables, but with insufficient proteins to service muscle mass, pose yet another type of challenge. Ultra-low carbohydrate diets are helpful in maintaining low weight levels but may pose challenges to sustaining daily energy levels. Proper portions of total caloric intake and of each type of food are critical to a diet that will maintain optimum health and fitness levels.

Modern wellness programs are centered on a balance of nutrients, particularly the proportion of proteins to carbohydrates in your diet. There are various recommendations as to the amounts of proteins versus carbohydrates, size of portions, time of day each type of nutrient is eaten, etc. These recommendations will depend on your overall wellness goals. For example, if you are seeking to build more strength and power, a higher protein loaded diet may be fitting. To build endurance, a diet more balanced in complex carbohydrates and limited in pure protein would be more fitting. If weight loss is a high priority, a diet centered on plant based nutrition is most appropriate.

As mentioned, many dietary guidelines are also now recommending eating several smaller meals throughout the day versus three traditional larger meals we have been accustomed to. These programs often recommend specific types of nutrients throughout the day to stimulate and maintain your metabolism, support the proper hypertrophy and recovery in your musculoskeletal system and to aid in more thorough digestion. What is best for you? Again, that depends upon your primary wellness goals. Research and plan your daily nutrition requirements as carefully as you can, then use self-discipline to execute that plan.

Your actual portion sizes should vary according to your body type, size, gender, age, targeted ideal weight and activity levels. For example, the amount of daily complex carbohydrate intake for a person training for a marathon should be much higher than for a bodybuilder or someone who is generally sedentary. The portions should fit the activity levels and metabolism. It may take a fair amount of research and experimentation to find the ideal calorie levels for your specific situation.

If you have a high metabolism and have difficulty putting on or maintaining muscle mass, you can probably safely consume more protein or carbohydrates on a daily basis than someone with a slow metabolism. If you have a body type with a slower metabolism or that easily and rapidly stores body fat, then total caloric intake, especially the amount of carbohydrate intake, should be carefully considered. Plant based diets may be more appropriate than even modest levels of protein or carbohydrates.

You should never eat until you feel overly full. Establishing habits of eating lesser amounts or until mildly comfortable is much healthier than bingeing on large amounts of food in a single sitting. Further, snacking is not necessarily a taboo. Healthy snacks, in proper portions, can be easily worked in to a wellness centered nutrition plan. Remember, the key to healthy eating is eating only the amounts and types of food your body can digest, process and use in your daily metabolic functioning and activities. It is a fine balance, but it can be achieved.

Your portion sizes determine the total amount of calories you consume in a day. As mentioned, you should eat according to your body type, overall size and weight and activity levels. There are numerous suggested ways to compose your daily calorie intake. A typical example of a useful calorie chart is shown below. As with any wellness principle, the more you research and learn the more equipped you are for success. Such charts are beginning guidelines, not hard and fast limits.

Average Calorie Intake Guide (May Vary)				
BODY WEIGHT	Male Sedentary	Male Active	Female Sedentary	Female Active
115-125lbs	1800	2000	1500	1700
125-140lbs	2000	2200	1600	1800
140-165lbs	2100	2400	1700	2000
165-200lbs	2200	2800	1700	2100
200-230lbs	2400	3000	1700	2200
230-260lbs	2600	3200	1800	2300
260 Plus lbs	2800	3300	2000	2400

Generic Calorie Chart

Whole Foods versus Processed Foods

One of the challenges we face with the modern American diet is, as one expert put it, "Eating more food like substances and less real food." The modern world seems to move according to a hurried schedule. The time to shop for, prepare, cook and eat whole foods is lacking in many of our daily routines. What is a whole food? It is a plant, meat, grain, fruit, vegetable or dairy that is as close to its natural state as possible.

Basically a whole food is a food that has not undergone any alteration due to a processing method such as canning, preserving, chemical alteration or cooking in certain ways. Raw vegetables such as a spinach or kale, whole grains that are unprocessed such as oatmeal or cracked wheat, raw nuts and fruits picked and naturally ripened are examples of whole foods. In the place of whole and natural foods it is easy to substitute processed and manufactured foods.

The stores of America are stocked full of processed foods. They are quick (if not always inexpensive) and easy to prepare and consume compared to whole foods. The problems with processed foods are numerous. First, processing foods often erodes the nutritional content of the food compared to its whole state. Second, numerous fillers, chemicals and other substitutes may be mixed in with the processed food that does not contribute in any way to nutrition or health and may actually be harmful with continued long term consumption. Third, the caloric values of processed foods are usually much more than equivalent whole foods. Fourth, while it remains a subject of further research and debate, the life or energy of whole foods may be lost in processing. And fifth, the amount of fiber in processed foods is often greatly reduced.

Fiber is the non-digestible roughage that is contained in many vegetables, legumes and grains that aids in digestion, hinders absorption of detrimental fats and helps clear out other undigested foods and contaminants in the digestive tract. Almost every nutrition expert recommends diets rich in fiber for positive nutritional and digestive health. Whole foods are usually richer in usable raw fiber than processed foods.

Another category of whole foods are organic foods. These are often more traditional foods such as meat, grains and vegetables that are grown without any artificial chemical, hormonal or other additives. Some unprocessed foods may still have additives such as growth hormones used to accelerate the growth and harvest cycles of animals. There is an increasing body of research that suggests ingestion of these additives in our foods may have harmful long term effects. Other considerations such as lack of pesticides to crops, certain soil conditions or natural types of feed may be used as criteria to label food as organic. Organic foods tend to be more expensive than their non-organic equivalents. The cost and health benefits of organic foods should at least merit consideration in a wellness oriented diet plan.

Any way you look at it, whole foods are more beneficial in your diet than processed foods. They are almost always more nutritious, less fattening and probably tastier as well. Yet, the love affair with processed and fast foods marches on. This is not to say that any fast food or processed food is innately harmful, but a diet that consists mainly of these types of "food like substances" as its staples may pose a serious health threat over time. An easy rule of thumb is to consume three parts raw food to any one part of processed foods that you eat. Remember that whole foods will almost always be healthier and more nutrient dense per calorie than any processed alternative.

Alternative Nutrition and Superfoods

Along with strides in the fields of general nutrition, there exists substantial research that suggests certain foods contain extraordinary nutritional values per consumed calorie. These foods are deemed "Superfoods" due to their natural ability to provide a superabundance of specific nutrients. While research continues to explore the actual benefits of many of these alternatives to traditional foods, there is plenty of anecdotal evidence as well as mounting scientific evidence to suggest that some foods are particularly effective in providing nutrient rich calories.

Other touted benefits of Superfoods are lower cholesterol, reduced body fat and boosts to immunity. Some of the more popular Superfoods being marketed today include: Goji, wheatgrass, acai, mangosteen, noni, pumpkin, papaya, barley, bean sprouts, spirulina, bee pollen, blue-green algae, royal jelly, maca, seaweed and many others.

As with any non-traditional nutritional sources, research the costs and benefits carefully. Determine what sounds attractive and what foods might contain the benefits you would personally seek in a complete nutrition plan. Beware of overzealous claims and miraculous benefits of one food or another. You can only benefit from carefully crafting alternative nutrition into an overall plan and vision for total nutritional fitness.

The Burgeoning Market of Supplementation

If there is one area of fitness that has literally exploded over the last decade it is the field of performance supplements. Supplementation no longer means just taking a daily multi-vitamin. There seems to be a supplement available for anything you can imagine. Strength, size, stamina, recovery, specific targeted nutrition, sleep and more are covered in the claims of the numerous products now available. There are many products even making claims to enhance the body on a genetic level. You could spend days, even weeks on end researching and cataloging the numerous supplements with their accompanying claims.

Supplements fall into two basic sub-categories. These are performance enhancers, such as protein drinks, energy drinks, creatine, pre-workout and post workout formulas, recovery products and so on. Another category includes nutritional enhancers such as vitamins, Aloe Vera, Echinacea, Ginseng, Gingko Biloba, Tea Tree Oil and other chemical or herbal products. Such supplements usually make specific claims as to their purpose and effect. You should research carefully any supplements usage and claims.

A majority of athletes and many fitness enthusiasts that train to perform at high levels use one or more supplementation products as part of their daily nutrition. Anecdotal evidence certainly suggests that many supplement products do deliver on their claims to some degree or another. But the truth is that some products may not, and some caution and care is recommended.

While there are many supplements that undoubtedly perform up to their specific claims, there may be others that are simply an expensive waste of time. Supplements can quite costly compared to whole foods. A simple rule for supplementation is to research products carefully, beware of extraordinary claims, integrate products into a complete nutritional plan and then self-monitor for results.

One developing and promising avenue for effective supplementation revolves around using bio-frequency technologies that can measure nutritional deficiencies in the body. Each individual tends to process nutrients in a slightly unique way. For example, if your hair greys early, it may be a result of a deficiency in processing copper. If your nails become brittle it may be associated with difficulty in absorbing calcium. There are emerging technologies that can identify these deficiencies and prescribe a specific mix of supplementation to counter them. Whatever your situation, supplements can be used to enhance good dietary habits. They may even boost performance to a degree. They are certainly not substitutes for a proper diet; they should be used in conjunction with a carefully structured, wellness oriented nutrition plan.

The Four White Poisons and Other Hazards

While there are many foods that need to be included in a proper nutrition plan, there are a few items that need to be monitored closely due to their potentially harmful effects on the human body. These are commonly termed the four white poisons: animal fat, processed sugars, salt and bleached white flour. Each one of these common substances has been found to have harmful effects on the body when consumed in significant amounts.

Fatty meats will raise cholesterol levels and contribute to unwanted body fat. Processed sugars are found in sweets such as soda, cookies, cake, ice cream and candy. These sugars spike the body's blood sugar levels requiring insulin for regulation. This is known as raising your body's glycemic index. Eating carbohydrate rich foods that constantly spike your glycemic index make weight control very difficult. Not only do these sugars stress your blood insulin levels, excess sugars are immediately stored in body fat. Research has linked processed sugars with a number of health, mental dysfunction, immunity and illness related problems, especially diabetes.

In addition to the common processed sugar, other forms of sugars have found their way into nearly every processed food. These take the form of corn syrup, fructose, sucrose and other refined sugars. These have equally deleterious effects when ingested in significant amounts. Many artificial sweeteners, such as aspartame, sorbitol or xylitol, while eliminating the calories of processed sugars may have other chemically related ill effects. Stevia, natural honey and agave have been shown to be much safer alternatives to sugar. Check the ingredients of processed foods carefully to see what type and how much of these sugars are contained therein.

Salt is necessary for many bodily functions, but in excess can lead to high blood pressure or gout. Bleached white flour is found in numerous processed foods and bread products. Bleached flour has many of the critical nutrients found in whole flours processed out. It also stresses blood sugar levels and contributes to unwanted weight gain. A wellness oriented diet should be designed around ingesting minimal amounts of foods containing these substances. While some more enthusiastic experts might counsel you to avoid these substances completely, moderation and balance is the key to success in most reasonable diet plans.

While the items listed above are the most commonly ingested compounds that can have an adverse effect on the body, they are not the only suspects that might infringe on your wellness and health. Excessive amounts of caffeine, alcohol or harmful drugs have no place in a personal wellness plan for obvious reasons. As with the compounds above, moderation is important.

Also be aware of other hidden dangers in many of the foods we eat, particularly processed foods. These hidden suspects are compounds known as saturated fats. These "cheap" fats have been linked to high cholesterol levels, obesity and even cancer. These substances can be found on food labels and go by titles such as palm kernel oil, cottonseed oil, coconut oil and palm oil. Less harmful are unsaturated fats such as olive oil, peanut oil, canola oil, corn oil, safflower oil and sunflower oil. The presence of these oils in almost all processed foods is reason enough to read food labels carefully. Avoid these fats when possible, but always remember the keys of balance and moderation in consuming foods containing these substances.

The volume by which these potentially harmful substances have been added to many of our processed foods reinforces the argument for a diet revolving around whole foods. For you to be successful in maintaining nutrition that supports wellness, you must be aware and study the ingredients and additives in the foods you eat. USDA labelling laws mandate that all of these elements be listed on food packaging. Study the foods you consume. Be responsible and always know what is in them.

The Importance of Hydration

The human body is made up primarily of water. For example, muscle fiber averages an 85% water content. Without constant ingestion of life giving liquids, your body will deteriorate, systems will shut down and you will die in a matter of days. It is not hyperbole to say that liquid intake is the single most important input into the complex machine that is the human body. You need sufficient hydration to make every other aspect of health and nutrition function. While proper hydration is arguably the most critical aspect of wellness, it is often one of the most overlooked. It is estimated that over half of all the people on this planet go through their day in a state of constant dehydration.

Water carries necessary oxygen to every part of the body. Every cell requires oxygen to function. Respiration is the main source of oxygenation in cells, but the oxygen content in water (H2O) is a very important secondary source of oxygen. Proper hydration keeps cells and organs healthy and working properly. Water carries nutrients throughout the body. It also cleanses the body at a cellular level and removes toxins. Proper hydration helps maintain healthy pH levels throughout the body and supports healthy neuro-electrical and neuro-chemical systems. In short, water is necessary for the healthy functioning of virtually every system in your body.

Most experts recommend between a half gallon and gallon of water be consumed each day to maintain proper hydration levels. The need for hydration increases with escalated activity levels due to loss of moisture through sweat and respiration. Liquids need to be consumed constantly. If you have a feeling of thirst, your body is already past a point of hydration deficit. If you feel thirsty, you need additional liquids to catch up to your body's needs.

An important issue surrounding your ability to hydrate is the nature and quality of liquids that you take into your body. While some hydration may be obtained from food, such as fresh fruit, the majority of your body's hydration will come from the liquids you drink. All liquids are not created equal in their ability to provide thorough hydration and oxygenation to support healthy bodily function. Each ounce of liquid you drink has a specific capacity to carry water and oxygen throughout your body.

Pure unprocessed waters have the highest beneficial values. This is water that has come from natural unprocessed ground sources. It is water that has not been through significant purification or filtration processes that alter the natural ionic energy and content of the water. Some bottled natural spring waters maintain this purity and energy, while water from local municipal sources or bottled water that had been heavily purified, chlorinated, filtered or processed have much less energy and much less capacity to hydrate the body in comparison.

A specific scientific measure of water's ability to cleanse and hydrate the body is known as Oxidation Reduction Potential (ORP). This is a measurement of water's ability to add oxygen molecules to a system and remove hydrogen molecules and toxins from the system. The higher the ORP (expressed in negative numbers), the more effectively water will hydrate and detoxify the body. The lower the Positive ORP (expressed in positive numbers), the less water will be effective. In fact some water may barely "break even" in terms of hydration. For example, municipal water high in chlorine may expend any ORP value it might have in removing the toxic chlorine contained in the water.

This implies that all waters are not indeed equal in their ability to hydrate the body. Waters with a higher ORP value are simply "wetter" than other less ionically fresh and active water. If the best possible hydration is a concern for you, research available water in your area. See if you can obtain information on ORP values. Higher ORP waters may come at a price. But it may well be a price worth paying if the highest degrees of hydration are important to your mode of complete wellness.

Natural juices that are taken straight from the fruit and not concentrated or heavily filtered also contain significant levels of hydrating capacity. However, the sugars and other caloric content of processed juices may counter some of their hydrating capacities. Engineered sports drinks are another source of hydration, but their overall hydrating effect depends upon the quality of source water and the combinations of other ingredients, often salts and sugars, that may subtract from their overall ability to hydrate (although the intent of many such drinks is to also deliver electrolytes into the body).

The least effective liquids to consume in terms of hydration are liquids that contain contaminants, chemicals or other ingredients that offset their hydration values. Among these are coffee, beer, carbonated sodas and processed juices. These liquids all contain substances that compromise the ability of their water content to effectively hydrate the body, such as sugar, salt, caffeine and alcohol. All of these substances are toxic to the body and need hydration to be removed.

Also, as briefly mentioned above, the majority of municipal water systems in America use chlorine, iodine or other chemical purifiers that degrade the hydration and oxygenation value of their water. In fact, some systems may have such an excess of chemicals or other toxins in their water that it actually creates a negative hydration effect to drink it. This occurs when the chemicals and particulates in the water require more than the entire hydrating value of the water itself to remove them from the body.

Keeping yourself hydrated is a daily vigil. You should always maintain the discipline necessary to keep your body properly hydrated and functioning smoothly. This means making conscious efforts to drink lots of liquids. If you take hydration seriously, it also means being careful as to the quality of liquids you ingest. Proper hydration will ensure that you maintain vigorous activities, help you recover thoroughly and keep your internal systems functioning smoothly. A well fed human machine also needs to be properly lubricated with quality liquids.

Learn to Listen to Your Body

One of the great benefits of wellness is that it helps put you in closer touch with your own physical and mental constitution. Consistent application of wellness principles will more effectively develop your physical functions, but this discipline carries over to nurturing emotional and spiritual functions as well. Nutrition is certainly an important aspect of your whole self that wellness helps you refine. As you progress in your journey of personal wellness you will begin to sense your body's wants and needs with greater clarity.

As your levels of wellness increase, cravings for unhealthy foods will decrease and you will begin to intuitively perceive what your body needs to replenish, nourish and rebuild from day to day. You will sense when your body wants more protein or carbohydrates. You will naturally hydrate yourself at intervals when your body most needs it. You will find yourself drawn to healthy menu choices, healthy grocery lists and proper portions and varieties of foods.

As you achieve higher levels of wellness, you will realize a mental synergy and unity in catering to your daily nutritional needs. Remember that your body needs proper nutrition to function. Low calorie or fad diets are not generally effective. You need to feed your body consistently with proper amounts and variety. If you are thoughtful and sensitive, your body will help you understand what it needs and how much it needs. It will "speak" to your mental and spiritual sides. Learn to listen and respond accordingly.

This still does not relieve you from doing some homework. Learn about varieties of healthy foods. Research the many products and claims surrounding supplements. Read food labels to identify potential harmful ingredients. Sample a variety of whole and organic foods to see what fits your tastes. Avoid substances that may have addictive properties. Educate yourself as best you can then let your body help you understand the rest. The more you keep the garbage out of your body, the more you build long term wellness into it.

Quick Tips to Feed and Hydrate Your Machine

- Carry a water bottle with you throughout the day. Drink at least half a gallon of water in addition to other liquids.
- If you have any suspicions as to the quality of your municipal water, invest in a high level filtration system. Only drink filtered water or natural spring water.
- Incorporate water into your diet that originates from natural springs and has not been processed or filtered. Drink as much of this "virgin" water as you can afford.
- Make sure bottled water containers do not contain unhealthy levels of bisphenol A (BPA) or phthalate that are unhealthy to ingest.
- Visit a local health food store and consult with an in-house nutritionist as to specific health products and organic foods that fit a wellness based diet plan.
- Beware of "fruit juices" that are mostly water and sugars. Drink only natural 100% juices.
- Take a cooking class that focuses on lean and healthy cuisine choices.
- Learn to read the labels on all food you purchase. Avoid products that contain unacceptable levels of saturated fats and fillers.

- Learn portion control. A portion is roughly the amount you could hold in the palm of your hand, not an amount that takes up your plate. Use Apps or online resources to study portion size.
- When eating at restaurants, ask for a box to take part of your meal home with you. Immediately put a portion of your food in the box and eat it another day.
- When possible, shop for organic foods that are free of hormones or pesticides.
- Incorporate fresh raw foods such as fruits and uncooked vegetables into your diet daily.
- If you cannot avoid sweets, try dark chocolate with at least 60% Cacao. It is rich in anti-oxidants.
- Research diet alternatives through books or the internet. Based on your body type, buy only foods that meet your protein/carbohydrate/fiber requirements.
- Use smart phone or computer applications such as Diet Point or Addidas Mi Coach to outline calorie and diet parameters.
- Always eat whole grains versus products with bleached white flour.
- Limit the amount of meat in your diet. Look to incorporate nuts, seeds and legumes as a protein alternative.
- Limit your intake of coffee, tea, soda and alcoholic beverages as these will actually contribute to dehydration.
- Be specific with your supplementation. Target supplements that address a particular fitness need. Research your chosen supplements for established effects and anecdotal support.

REST AND RECOVERY ARE AN IMPORTANT PART OF OVERALL WELLNESS.

What happens in the time between periods of activity is every bit as important as the activity itself. Your body is indeed a marvelous biological machine. Just as high performing machines such as jet planes or race cars need regular and periodic maintenance, your body also needs frequent "down time." The vigorous movement involved with exercise activities breaks down muscle fibers and other soft tissues. It is the breaking down of the body physically and chemically, and then building it back up to a higher level, that increases overall fitness. This is the natural process your body goes through to increase its strength and stamina, maintaining hypertrophy.

Therefore, how you rest and recover has equally important implications to your health as the actual activities that produced fatigue in the first place. A fast paced modern lifestyle, with its subsequent stresses and pressures, only adds to the burdens that your body must recover from. There are many good people who live day to day in a state of perpetual exhaustion. It is crucial that you find the time to rest and to heal your body from the strains of the day, whether you have incurred them yourself through vigorous exercise or had them imposed upon you by external circumstances.

The Value of a Good Night's Sleep

Culturally, Americans have traditionally viewed sleep as a bit of a luxury. We have revered the person who sleeps little and works a lot to get ahead in the world. Benjamin Franklin coined the phrase "Early to bed and early to rise makes a man healthy, wealthy, and wise." Most of us probably have to rise early, especially if a daily exercise plan is involved. It is the early to bed part we tend to have a problem with.

Your body needs adequate sleep. For most normal individuals that is at least six and a half to seven hours per night. If you have stressed your body more than normal, you may need more than seven hours. As with your diet, listen to your body. Sleep patterns are one of the most natural biological rhythms you can master if you pay attention to what your body tells you. It is in the deep rhythmic patterns of sleep that your body rebuilds itself.

All sleep is not created equal. While a quick nap may energize you on a Sunday afternoon, it is deep, R.E.M. sleep that is required for your body to adequately recover and rebuild itself. R.E.M. (rapid eye movement) sleep is a deep state of sleep where there are certain high neurological functions paired with almost complete lack of muscle movement. Research indicates that the majority of physical recovery is accomplished during R.E.M. sleep. R.E.M. sleep is also associated with developing neuron pathways throughout the brain, nurturing the mind as well as the musculature.

You should experience three to five periods of R.E.M. sleep in a typical six to eight hour night. These sleep periods comprise only about two hours of your total sleep time, but are believed to encompass the majority of your recovery time. Since R.E.M. is a deeper state of sleep, it is important to maintain an environment that allows you to achieve these states throughout the night. Light, sound or other external interruptions should be minimized or eliminated. It is critical you structure and maintain an environment that is conducive to uninterrupted R.E.M. sleep.

Research suggests that individuals who do not achieve regular R.E. M. sleep cycles are open to a number of physical and psychological maladies. If you are not getting the proper rest, you will find regular vigorous activity difficult as inadequate recovery periods create strength and energy deficits.

It is also critical to have your body prepared for sleep when you are ready to go to bed. You should finish any meals or snacking several hours before you retire at night. Alcohol and caffeine ingested close to your bedtime may prevent your body from achieving the deeper states of sleep necessary for recovery.

Processing agitating, high level information or stimuli, such as reading technical literature, watching a horror movie, perusing a disturbing story on the internet or stressing about work or family issues just prior to sleep may also keep your mind engaged for some time after falling asleep, thus preventing the proper R.E.M. cycles. Preparing for and budgeting enough time for regular deep sleep is crucial to your strength, recovery, health and ultimately your sanity.

Nutrition and Physical Recovery

As mentioned in Pathway #8, proper nutrition is a key to adequate recovery and strength. Eating the right combination of proteins and carbohydrates, and ensuring adequate amounts of plant based foods rich in vitamins and minerals are an important part of your body's ability to recover. All the sleep in the world will not be helpful if your body has not been stocked with the nutrients necessary to rebuild muscles, bones, organs and tissues. One of the downsides of harmful substances, such as excessive caffeine, alcohol or drug consumption, is that they not only hinder the absorption of healthy nutrients, but lessen the body's ability to recover and heal itself.

Eating large meals or taking powerful supplements such as performance-enhancing herbs or vitamins close to bedtime may also elevate your metabolism at a time of day when you should be allowing your metabolism to wind down. Eating well with proper nutrition on a descending schedule is the key to good recovery. Solid meals in the morning followed by the largest food intake from noon to three, tapering off with smaller meals in the evening will help your body prepare for a strong recovery overnight.

There are many strategies for supplementation, including natural and herbal supplements, doctor supervised steroid therapy and growth hormones, which are geared toward increasing your recovery ability. While research suggests that many such methods may shorten or enhance recovery times, they may trigger dangerous side effects and are not a substitute for proper rest and recovery. Greatly enhancing the body's recovery through unnatural means in order to work even harder may yield short to medium term gains in strength and fitness, but pose long term risks to overall wellness and physiological balance.

The Hazards of Overactivity

For dynamic and aggressive athletes and wellness enthusiasts who participate in significant and consistent activities, one of the problems that may be encountered is the phenomenon known as overtraining. This occurs when the cumulative sum of your physical activities begin to outpace your body's natural ability to recover. It is easily possible, particularly for more well-conditioned individuals, to work their bodies harder than their ability to rest and recover before their next activity.

The symptoms of overtraining are a decrease in performance coupled with an increased risk of injury. If your body's tissues are being torn down through consistent strenuous activity, and then are not rebuilt through proper nutrition and rest, the likelihood you will have over-stressed joints or muscles break down is greatly increased.

It is actually easier than you might imagine to reach your body's absolute maximum capacity for strenuous activity. This is particularly true as you age. Age subsequently brings reduced recovery ability. You may have the ideal routines, the perfect nutrition plan and the best supplements on the market, but with time comes diminishing capacity, particularly when it comes to your body's ability to recover. At age fifty, you might be able to do the things you did at thirty once in a while, but if you keep subjecting your body to such strenuous activities on a daily basis you will pay a steep price and may be heading for a breakdown and possibly injury.

The solution to overtraining is simple. Take it down a notch. Take a week off. Take the pedal off the metal for a while. Most fitness experts recommend that you take at least two weeks per year with no stressful physical activity. These down times are critical for complete rest and recovery of joints and muscles. As you age, it may be necessary to schedule four weekly respites per year.

If you do not feel that you want take time off, lighten up the routines you are doing. Schedule "light days" into your routine where you do exercises of reduced intensity. Whatever you do, build in time for proper recovery. Your body needs it. It will keep you fresh and motivated and less prone to injury.

Alternative Recovery and Healing Methods

Outside of deep, restful sleep and the proper nutrition, there are other methods that have benefit to enhanced recovery of the body. There exists a wide variety of treatments and therapies designed to accentuate and enhance the healing of the body. Many of these methods have accumulated clinical evidence of their effectiveness, while others are purely anecdotal.

Whatever types of recovery treatment you might find interesting or helpful, many of these enhanced methods become a matter of preference, time and affordability. Alternative healing is often age related. The older you get the longer it takes for your body to recover. If you are very active into your forties, fifties and beyond, the field of alternative recovery becomes more relevant and appealing.

Enhanced recovery methods that may appeal to a person in their forties are probably not under consideration for an active person in their twenties, simply because of a lack of perceived necessity or benefit. Some of the most popular methods of alternative recovery include massage therapy, heat and cold treatments, acupressure, detoxification wraps and soaks, compression garments, magnetic field therapy, hydrotherapy, oxygen therapy, meditation and many others.

Alternative recovery methods are focused on specific therapies used to enhance the body's innate healing abilities. For example, deep tissue sports massage is one discipline that focuses on aligning, smoothing and detoxifying the muscle tissues throughout the body. The specific manipulations of massage have been shown to relax and heal muscles more rapidly than if the tissues were left to their own physiological processes. Many massage disciplines have a proven record of enhancing healing and recovery and preventing injury in sports applications. Massage has gained momentum in its many disciplines as one of the most popular alternative therapies available today.

Other methods, such as detoxifying herbal wraps, are designed to draw out toxins from body tissues which might inhibit the natural recovery and healing processes. Therapies employing heat and cold, using such traditional tools as ice bags and hot tubs, have been a staple of trainers for decades. Other disciplines, such as magnetic field therapy and healing frequency therapy are more experimental and are still accumulating useful research and anecdotal data.

However you feel about your physical state on a daily basis, always stay closely in tune with your body's recovery cycles. As with principles in other Pathways, learn to listen to your body. It will let you know when it is well rested and when it needs help in this area. Constant nagging pain or injury is one sign that proper recovery is not being realized. If you are constantly relying on stimulants to maintain daily energy levels, you may conclude that greater recovery strategies are necessary.

If you feel tired, run down or lack energy and enthusiasm in any of your activities, take a hard look at your recovery times between those activities. There are times throughout a week, month or year when doing less may result in achieving more sustainable wellness long term. Your best exercise or activities will not have the desired effect if your body has not recovered from previous activities. Always incorporate the time intervals necessary in your fitness plan to allow proper rest and recovery.

Additionally, we all need a time for mental and spiritual recovery. Stress levels and constant tracking and processing of necessary information in a complex modern world tend to wear on us mentally. We may suffer "burnout" or other forms of mental fatigue. Alternative recovery methods, though not always clinically proven, show great merit when combatting this type of weariness.

Meditation, as manifest through prayer, Chakra, Yogi or Zen meditation, has shown great benefit in refreshing mind and spirit. More will be written about this Pathway #12. Finding a place of peace, rest and contemplation can be a necessity in a busy world and busy life. Finding emotional space to recover from constant stress and activity, even beneficial activity, is crucial. Everyone needs to "unstring the bow" and "sharpen the saw" with regularity. The key is identifying your calming space and methodology.

Quick Tips for Rest and Recovery

- Rest does not always mean going into "couch potato" mode. Healthy and non-strenuous recreation, such as taking a walk, playing a board game with your friends or stargazing can help you recover as well.
- Make sure you do not eat at least two to three hours before retiring at night. An overworked digestive system will inhibit the necessary R.E.M. sleep you need.
- If your body feels tired, change your routine of activities to incorporate light days or days off until you feel able to work hard on a consistent basis.
- Try to sleep at least six to seven hours every night. Short weekday sleep periods punctuated by long weekend sleep periods are not as effective.
- Check your sleeping area for light and sound. Dark and quiet yield deeper sleep and less external interruption.

- Take a meditation class alone or with friends. Learn to relax yourself in any environment or situation.
- Experiment with massage therapy, detoxifying body wraps, magnetic field therapy, crystal therapy and other alternative methods of body healing. See if anything works for you to help you recover more thoroughly.

EMOTIONAL WELLNESS; ATTITUDE INFLUENCES WELLNESS ALTITUDE.

At its core, wellness is an emotional commitment. What is the basis for emotional wellness? It involves cutting through the noise of daily living and focusing on concepts, feelings, activities and desires that comprise a positive outlook. In other words, emotional wellness is about forming realistic and positive attitudes. To be emotionally well you must be able to focus on the positive and beneficial aspects of daily living and mitigate the negative influences and events you will inevitably encounter. You must find the strength to create positivity.

You can begin by asking yourself what you really think about the whole idea of personal fitness and overall wellness. Does it sound attractive to you? Is the broader philosophy of wellness paramount to how you envision living a full, healthy and fulfilled life? Does activity centered wellness sound burdensome or overwhelming? Is it such a low priority with everything else going on in your life that you see it as something you will get around to eventually, if you find the time? Can you make the connection between your decisions for a wellness oriented lifestyle and the overall quality of your lifestyle?

Do you see your personal wellness as something that you truly have control over, or is it subject to circumstances beyond your control? How you answer these questions frames the truth you face in an honest self-assessment. If there is one thing you can change more quickly than your own levels of wellness, it is your attitude toward wellness and toward yourself. Your positive assessment and acceptance of your self-image and the attitudes you create will motivate you to achieve greater personal wellness and enhance your overall state of being.

A Hierarchy of Emotional Wellness Perspective and Attitude

Your emotional perspective and attitudes are framed and dictated by the perspective you have about any specific subject. When it comes to wellness, the more you know, the more equipped you are to make decisions that will be beneficial to you. When it comes to wellness, there are no wrong answers that may inhibit you, just bad information and limiting assumptions. The whole point of this book is to point you in the direction of good and useful information and assist you in making positive and beneficial assumptions about yourself and your true state of wellness.

To assist in this process, it helps to understand where you are in the hierarchy of emotional wellness perspective and attitude. Since attitude determines altitude, or the length to which you may achieve in any endeavor, you should be honest with yourself in assessing your own commitment to a wellness lifestyle. These levels are illustrated as follows:

Level 1 – Blind Conformance: You perform wellness activities at the behest of others. It is family or peer group pressure that keeps you engaged, when you decide to engage. At this level there is no driving personal philosophy that would keep you engaged. Your attitude is equally geared towards avoidance as engagement with no long term vision.

Level 2 – Avoiding Consequence: You perform wellness activities to avoid negative consequences that you view as harmful. You will remain engaged as long as the negative consequence is held at bay. Your attitude is driven by fear of a negative outcome as opposed to a positive mindset. You see primarily short term outcomes.

Level 3 – External Reward: You engage is wellness activities that bring a perceived external reward. Perhaps this is the recognition and praise of other, or a financial prize in a group challenge at work. Perhaps it is the reward of a more positive self-image. Your attitude is geared toward the acquisition of the reward and what it represents to you. Your vision extends as far as the meaning of the reward.

Level 4 – Vision Driven: You engage in wellness in response to a well-informed personal vision, advised by study and experimentation. You associate wellness activities with a long-term perspective of benefits and positive lifestyle results. Your attitude is one of enjoyment and engagement with a clear correlation of activities and results.

Level 5 – Internalization: You consistently engage in wellness because that is who you are at your core. You feel a lifestyle revolving around wellness is your natural state of being. Your attitude is one of both desiring to live according to the tenets of wellness and sharing the fruits of wellness with others.

Where do you feel that you are personally within this framework? What do you need to learn and do to be able to internalize wellness and create within yourself an attitude placing wellness as a top priority? Do you understand that time and experience will reinforce the benefits of wellness and you will naturally ascend these levels based on consistent and beneficial outcomes?

And indeed that is the natural ascending course of a wellness oriented lifestyle. Your positive attitude towards wellness will be reinforced through correct and consistent activity that elevates your entire life. You will experience personal benefits manifest in greater health, less illness, greater productivity, greater mental and spiritual capacity, enhanced economic success, stronger relationships and many other positive outcomes.

Base Your Attitude on Realistic Expectations, not Comparison with Others

One of the great challenges of living in a society with constant media bombardment is that we daily receive images of individuals that have achieved their physical ideals and top professional success. These images gracing our magazines, personal devices and televisions are often celebrities, sports figures or fitness gurus that have, through painstaking work and professional guidance, maximized their personal physical potential. It is a natural inclination to compare yourself to others. This is a misdirected and often unhealthy way to think of yourself.

One cannot see the weeks and months of personal training, professional dieticians, paid exercise time, painstaking professional makeup or even the photo airbrushing that result in these idealized images that are paraded in front of us so regularly. The most important comparison you can make is to compare yourself now to yourself at some point in the past. Further, you should realistically assess where you are now in the Hierarchy of Wellness and establish a vision of what you wish to become in the future.

Forming a healthy attitude about yourself has no foundation or bearing in the achievements of anyone else. It requires a strict focus on your own desires and expectations. Negative or unrealistic attitudes toward yourself, your self-image, or misleading thoughts that you cannot improve yourself and your life through greater wellness will defeat you before you even begin. If you are constantly sending yourself negative messages and seeing the downside of physical activity or the lack thereof, you hamper your own ability to grow and improve.

Always remain positive and stay within yourself. Learn what works best for you and stick with it. Know your preferences, understand your genetic composition and your own strengths and limitations. Understanding all of these allows you to maintain positive attitude by keeping your progress within the bounds of your own personal framework.

Attitudes can be Transformational

Attitude goes beyond feeling positive about doing something to better yourself. The improving physical image you see in the mirror only goes so far towards reinforcing your attitudes regarding overall wellness. Ego driven results or results based on short term criteria are shallow and temporary in their satisfaction and are not sustainable for longer periods of time or throughout various life phases. Your attitude is formed and nurtured through consistent application of proper principles translated into action continued over time.

Your attitude toward wellness has the capability to transform you completely over time. If you maintain a positive attitude toward your goals, plans, programs and activities not only will you look better and feel better, you will become a richer and more complete individual. This growth and individual development is a natural consequence of positively and consistently applying wellness principles.

The self-discipline and self-mastery that comes with regular application of personal wellness will reinforce other positive attitudes and aspects you deem important. You will not just feel that you are in control of yourself, you will know that you are in control. The principled foundation of achieving a high degree of wellness reinforces attitudes of confidence and success in other pursuits. You will feel more confident in your work, your love life, your intellectual interests, your spiritual commitments and your social endeavors. The attitudes that you develop necessary to remain engaged in a long-term wellness lifestyle contribute to a mindset of confidence and success for any other relevant aspect of your life.

The principles encompassed within the Twelve Pathways are time-tested and proven to elevate your personal levels of wellness if they are correctly applied. The application of these or any other principle begins with a desire to apply such principles. You have to really want it and do what it takes to achieve it. The results that you harvest by consistent application of these principles will continue to reinforce and shape a positive attitude and self-image.

A positive attitude toward your fitness potential leads to positive actions that will engender positive results. This self-reinforcing cycle from attitude to results is central to a sustained effort to increase and maintain personal fitness. When it comes to wellness, your thoughts and realistic visions of a fitter, more complete you can be fulfilled as long as you maintain a positive and dynamic attitude. If you desire it enough, if you discipline yourself and your time in ways that will make it happen, you can and will achieve your wellness goals. It all starts with desire. Desire feeds an attitude of action. Action directed by correct principles and practices will get positive results. These are the building blocks in a foundation of a wellness centered life. It really is that simple.

Quick Tips to Maintain Positive Attitude

- A thousand mile journey begins with a single step. Always celebrate the little achievements, and keep going one day at a time.
- Realistic expectations bring realistic results and personal satisfaction. Raise your sights, but keep your vision at a level you can reach.
- Remember that the direction you face is what counts. Always picture yourself moving forward, and feel confident you can reverse direction if you are moving back.
- Take an unbiased inventory of your body type and perceived strengths and weaknesses. Design activities to your strengths and avoid your weaknesses.
- Always keep in mind that your increased personal wellness does not only benefit you, but everyone who is important to you.
- Always seek to surround yourself with like-minded individuals. Optimism is contagious; but so is discouragement. It is difficult to soar like an eagle if you are surrounded by turkeys.
- View challenges to your wellness goals as opportunities. Make a specific plan to overcome each challenge.

- Realistically envision yourself as the person you want to eventually become. Keep on striving and raising your sights. Reward yourself for significant achievements.
- Records create a referable history. Keep track of wellness goals such as weight, progress in activities and other important parameters. Refer back to these records periodically to check and reinforce your progress.

NURTURE YOUR POSITIVE INTELLECTUAL, SOCIAL, AND SPIRITUAL PASSIONS

The concept of wellness only begins with a healthy physique and efficiently functioning bodily systems. Wellness encompasses the intellectual and spiritual parts of your being every bit as much or more than it does the physical side of your nature. The mind, spirit and body are united in mysterious and profound ways to form the magnificent creature we call a human being. These separately identifiable but inextricably linked aspects of your constitution must work well together and in their respective operations to engender overall wellness.

Further, how you extend yourself and nurture yourself socially through positive relationships is a significant part of overall wellness. To truly live a wellness lifestyle suggests associating with other like-minded individuals as well as being a good example of what a complete and well person should be like.

Illness of the body can inhibit the mind and spirit. A diseased mind can seriously adversely affect the body and spirit. A depressed or empty spirit can easily offset any physical or intellectual gain. Caustic or unsupportive relationships can bring sorrow and stress. Wellness begins with an internal balance. It is best described as fitness of all parts of your being and healthy activities throughout all aspects of your life. A healthy body is at its best when it is the domain of a well fed mind and spirit also.

The Mind and Spirit can be Fed and Exercised

How do you see yourself? Are you in touch with the more esoteric aspects of your own being? Do you value intellectual pursuits at least as much as physical ones? Are you spiritually in tune with your own emotions and the wants and needs of those around you? Are you the person you want to be in the company of others? Can you show leadership when you need to and humility and gratitude for the talents of others when appropriate? Fine tuning your own self-perception to accurately match the realities that you face each day and the wellness goals you strive for is important.

Just as your body is programmed to always respond to exercise in adequate amounts, so your mind and intellect will respond to uplifting stimulation. One of the most profound aspects of your intelligence is that it is always active, always searching for something new to learn; something interesting to absorb and integrate into your understanding. From a purely intellectual perspective, your entire life could be described as the summation of all of the cerebral input you receive, information you absorb and the learning processes you undertake. It naturally follows that part of your total wellness should include keeping your mind active, sharp and always on the path to greater learning and knowledge.

If there is one general rule that overshadows all others in this age of information, it is the fact that there is more information now available to you than you could absorb in several lifetimes. It is impossible to be an expert at all things, and fairly difficult to be an expert at even a few things. To become an expert in even one field of significant human endeavor often requires years, if not a lifetime, of dedicated work, learning and discipline. There is simply so much information available, so much you could possibly learn.

Satisfying your intellect simply requires you to find something for which you have an interest and develop it into a passion for learning. Feed your mind constantly with useful and mind-expanding information; knowledge that contributes to a more complete understanding of yourself and the world around you. Your intellectual pursuits might be part of a career or they may be simply a hobby that keeps you centered and gives you joyful relief from the stresses and strains of the day. Whatever your interests, make sure to include information and learning that is more than the trivial. Just as a steady diet of cheese fries and pork rinds will not fuel your body for healthy and strong activity, a constant ingestion of comedy movies and celebrity gossip magazines will not deepen your intellect.

What are the relevant subjects that fascinate you? Astronomy, paleontology, chess, geology, holistic medicine, history, current events, art, politics, bridge, community service, gourmet cooking, agriculture, or genealogy? Nearly everyone has something that "turns them on" intellectually. What is your fascination? Do you devote time regularly to increase your understanding and knowledge of your favorite subjects? Do you feel a desire to continually learn and store useful information?

Do you regularly engage in activities that provide you with new and interesting stimuli? Do you feel empowered when you recognize that your base of understanding can and will broaden, expand and increase as you apply yourself to learning and retaining various fields of knowledge? If so, you are well on your way to sustaining wellness of your mind as well as your body. Do you feel inspired to share your discoveries and passions with others? Do you actively seek to associate with such like-minded individuals? Shared passions make for strong and productive relationships.

The same dynamics apply to your spiritual nature. For the sake of discussion, your spiritual nature is identified as that part of you that rises above the obvious daily routines and activities. It is that part of you that senses you are greater than just the sum of your biological existence. It is the center of your nature when considering the metaphysical possibilities that lay just behind and beyond your daily experiences. Spirituality can be centered on the idea or concept of deity, of a being or power beyond the ordinary or mortal. It can be centered on a concept of divine nature, a sense of self that rises above the physical needs. It can be based upon a feeling of unity with greater energy and forces that seem to permeate our world on a different level or plane. It can simply be a higher association with the natural world and the perceived force or energy that surrounds you. However you define your own personal spiritual nature, you need to feed and nurture that part of you also.

Intrinsic in the idea of spirituality is the notion that there are values to uphold and ethical ways to conduct yourself. Just as you must discipline yourself according to certain principles to achieve higher levels of physical wellness, so you must conform your actions and thoughts toward the ideals that your personal levels of spirituality suggest. You cannot be hypocritical in achieving physical conditioning. You cannot truthfully tell yourself that by skipping the necessary mileage you have designed to run in a week that you will become more aerobically fit. It simply will not happen. Neither should you sell yourself short on nurturing the activities that can enlarge your sense of spiritual well-being. You need to feed your spirit frequently, just as you feed your mind and body.

Do you consistently and periodically feel that you are a part of something larger than yourself? Do you explore ideas of religion, spiritualism and other metaphysical concepts with a true and pure intent to increase your understanding? Have you internalized a moral code that you feel can guide you in ways that are consistent with living in harmony with others and the world around you? Do you honestly strive to live each day according to that code as you best can understand and apply it?

Intellectual and Spiritual Wellness Impact Social Health

How does the sharpening of your intellectual and spiritual qualities affect your relationships? Do you spend your time associating with people who can lift you and also be uplifted by you? Are the bulk of your relationships healthy and mutually contributive versus needy, draining and counterproductive? Can you see the faults in others and not condemn them for their faults, but seek to lift them? Can you easily see and correct your own faults when they become apparent? All of these characteristics are important to being socially well.

Do you feel a personal sense of satisfaction when you can retire each day sensing you have done your best to make the people and the world around you a little better than when the day began? Do you frequently look for new ideas that can expand and contribute to a greater understanding of your spiritual nature and the nature of others around you? Any one or a combination of these key questions can lead you down a path to greater spiritual and social understanding and contribute to a real sense of personal growth and enlightenment. An active mind and enlightened spirit can only enhance the pursuits of your physical and social well-being. These synergies are always in play; they act upon you and those around you. You may truly find completeness in the sum of these separate but important parts.

The title of this section also notes that you should nurture positive intellectual, social and spiritual passions. Reflecting on some of the questions in this Pathway should bring to mind the concept of positive or beneficial growth in each of these aspects. This growth also functions on the principle of ingesting helpful and uplifting information. Continuing to study and test each aspect in your life should lead you to correct and helpful information, proper principles, actions and activities. It is in the activities you choose that wellness can be manifest, Choose healthy, stimulating and uplifting pursuits in each of these three areas.

Contract versus Covenant Relationships

Wellness is not a solo sport. We are intrinsically all linked in a commonality of human family. We will form relationships with hundreds if not thousands, of people over our lifetime. The type of relationships we are able to form can fall into two identifiable categories. One type of relationship is a contract relationship while another, a higher and more committed involvement, can be called a covenant relationship. To be truly well, these relationships need to be transacted on an appropriate basis.

A contract relationship is defined as a relationship between individuals based on an expectation or outcome from each other. It is in a sense "the art of the relationship deal". People with whom we have a contract relationship are individuals with whom we may contract business, join in a charitable cause or support a local institution or team. We enter the relationship with the idea we each will get what we want out of the relationship.

Healthy contract relationships are fine for casual or professional associations. You may know the local mailman, and as long as the mail gets delivered on time everything is fine. You may have a relationship with a junior league football coach who has your child on his team. There may be expectations associated with the relationship and as long as the coach meets those expectations, the relationship remains healthy.

Contractual relationships can be appropriate for interactions that do not need to get too personal, and can be kept at a transactive or professional level. When it comes to more personal, close and familial relationships, keeping a relationship at a contract level may not be appropriate. This is where it is crucial to learn and apply covenant relationships.

A covenant is a two way promise. Within the scope of relationships it is a promise between parties to mutually nurture and encourage the best in each other. What is obtained from the relationship, the transactional expectations, are subordinate to the overall positive becoming of each other. It is in this higher understanding of relationships that the most satisfying social satisfaction occurs.

It is the covenant based dedication to one another, with the patience, faith and sacrifice that may entail, that brings the most fulfillment. When it comes to social wellness, the greatest resource available is each other. If we recognize the need for covenant level commitments in our most important relationships, we will find more social strength, belonging and overall wellness. In a covenant relationship, the development of others is held at equal value to our own positive and wellness based progress.

The key is to instinctively understand where contract relationships are appropriate and where covenant relationships are necessary. For example, a marriage based strictly on the expectations of a contract relationship may head south quickly should those expectations not be upheld. Conversely, there may be no need for a covenant relationship and its deeper commitments with someone who runs a local restaurant. A cordial contractual interaction works just fine.

As with every other aspect of wellness, balance is always important. All aspects of self are equally critical to achieve overall wellness. Where you see the need to place emphasis is a highly personal decision. The key is not to let one aspect fall into neglect to service other aspects. Your emphasis may very well be determined by your personal situation. Whatever that situation is, think critically and clearly about how each of these areas of your life can be enriched.

And enrichment is the ultimate objective. While the physical aspects of wellness can be measured in concrete numbers, such as body mass, mile times or bench press weight, the intellectual, social and spiritual sides are much more subjective. How do you feel about your ability to grow intellectually, socially and spiritually? Are there barriers that prevent you from envisioning growth in these areas?

Feel confident you can and will develop each of these aspects of self with proper time and consistent application of activities that enrich mind and spirit. That heightened sense of self will surely grow, just as your physical growth follows appropriate physical activity. The maturity of each of these aspects of self define the core of complete wellness.

Quick Tips to Nurturing Your Intellectual, Social and Spiritual Passions

- Join a book-of-the-month club. Make a goal to read a new book each month. Vary the subjects of your books between informative and entertaining.
- Google a subject about which you have curiosity. See if you can find a dozen resources that provide useful information that increases your knowledge of that subject.

- Start a blog about something you have a passion for. Share ideas with other like-minded individuals.
- Write a paper on a subject you think is relevant or important at the moment. Give the paper to three friends and ask for their comments on the subject.
- Write a newspaper editorial on a current event you find particularly moving. Just for fun, send it in to a local paper and see if they will print it.
- Listen to beautiful music at least a few times a week. Identify music that makes you feel uplifted or energetic.
- Take music lessons to develop your musical talent. Choose an instrument you may have played earlier in life or try a new one.
- Plan trips to museums that display art, history, science and other interesting subjects. Plan field trips or "double dates" with other individuals with similar interests.
- Look for ways to be active in your local religious congregation. Search for opportunities to get outside of yourself and do something for others. Enjoy the internal rewards you feel from such service.
- Join a local bridge group. Read up on strategies to better play the game.
- Sharpen your word skills with a daily crossword puzzle and your logic skills with a daily Sudoku puzzle.
- Look for community service opportunities. Work with a local charity or homeless shelter. Seek service in others to expand the compassion within yourself.
- Find the beauty in others. Always look for a way to make someone else feel better about themselves. In so doing, you will feel better about your own place in the world.
- Have a "night out" with friends at least once a month. Plan creative group dates.

POSITIVE RENEWAL; FIND YOUR QUIET PLACE

At the end of each day you must be able to have a way to let all of the systems of your machine wind down and rebuild for the next day. As hard as a good activity based wellness program pushes you to increase your conditioning, so must there be a place and a time that you can simply relax and unwind, even if only for a while. Again, just like an automobile or airplane needs to be parked and maintained periodically, so your body needs that down time from strenuous activity. This is best achieved by finding an effective and convenient method to renew. Finding your own quiet place to effect that renewal amid the hectic days and weeks that comprise a well and fully lived life is a key principle to attaining personal wellness.

If you are disciplined enough to wind yourself up through vigorous activity, you must also be able to wind yourself down with regularity. There are also times in a given year that you should relax and allow your body to heal and recover for an extended period. You generally take a few weeks a year away from earning a living to vacation and relax. Likewise, many experts recommend a minimum of two one-week-long respites per calendar year free from stressful activity to allow rest and recovery of your muscles and joints.

Finding your quiet place is more than identifying a physical location where you are comfortable relaxing and allowing your cares to melt away and your body to rebuild. It is a state of mind that you can achieve through mental and spiritual discipline that allows you to free yourself from negative or unwanted thoughts and influences that can drag you down. Stress is one of the most detrimental factors affecting wellness. As mentioned earlier, physical activity is one of the best ways to counter the daily stresses you may be carrying. But freeing your mind from difficult or negative thoughts is also tantamount to good health.

A physical location away from the noise and stresses of daily activity is helpful, even with a disciplined state of mind. It could be as simple as driving an uncongested road outside of the crush of daily traffic. It could be a favorite nature trail. It could be a rooftop with a breathtaking view of the city. It could be a basement "man cave" with décor and memorabilia that elicits fond memories. It could be wherever you can find a moment of peace. There are times, regardless of your state of mind, when it is important to identify and renew yourself in such a place.

Wherever you find your quiet place, allow it to be a place where the stresses you have carried may be disposed of. Your quiet place should be an environment where your thoughts can wander freely, where you feel comfortable praying, meditating, resting or pondering that which is important to you. It should be a place where you can recover, re-energize, refresh and recreate your mind, spirit and body.

Your quiet place may be somewhere that is exclusively your own, or it may be someplace you share with someone special and close to you. It may be in your own home or it may be in a place far away that you can actually travel to or keep in the forefront of your mind. It may be somewhere that you discover or it may be a place your family has known for generations.

Wherever your quiet place is, or wherever it might be found, visit your quiet place frequently.

Take the time to reflect, ponder and re-establish your priorities in life. Take occasion to be honest with yourself and how you are doing in the important aspects of your wellness goals as well as your life goals. Laugh with yourself and forgive yourself for all that you have failed to accomplish. Smile with yourself and resolve to accomplish more than you already have. Ponder your direction in life, re-evaluate your priorities.

Remember and be thankful for every privilege and blessing you have had, including the trials through which you have passed. Remember that nothing in your life that is worthwhile comes easily, but that an attitude of determination, a little wisdom and a bit of luck will see you through. And never forget to take the time to thank yourself for a job well done and revere those good people who have been an important part of helping you get there. All this and more is the privileged domicile of your quiet place. But above all, remember to enjoy the journey.

Finding Quiet for Varying Personality Types

The concept of "quiet" can vary from person to person depending on their personality type. There are numerous frameworks for personality, type "A" versus type "B", a Meyers-Briggs ESTJ versus INFP, a Taylor Hartmann Red versus Blue, White or Yellow. Your personality forms a unique lens through which you perceive wellness. Personality and wellness imply different strategies for similar results. Although the principle holds true, the way you might envision applying that principle can vary widely. This is true for the type of activities you choose, and how you distinguish the concept of unwinding.

If you are highly competitive type "A" personality, a quiet place may be somewhere that is bustling and has an interest that calms your mind, but does not involve direct engagement with the environment. If you are more relaxed, a quiet place may be on a beach somewhere where no one else is around. A more fiery personality might perceive a brisk walk through the woods as a quiet engagement. A softer personality might perceive painting with water colors along the side of a lake as necessary relaxation. The Coffee House that one sees as an ideal break might be the crowded melee that repels another. Quiet is as you perceive it.

Differing personality types perceive wellness in different ways. Competitive activity versus more relaxing yet beneficial activities are both constructive on their own merits. How you perceive the benefit to yourself is key. A type "A" personality may perceive their optimum pursuit would be to snap off sub seven minute miles with regularity. A less competitive personality might see a two hour mountain hike through inspiring scenery with a friend as equally stimulating. Both move the participant towards greater wellness, despite defining activities or relaxation differently. It is simply a matter of perception and degrees.

Understanding Solutions to Stress

As mentioned earlier, stress is one of the most detrimental barriers to achieving consistent and high degrees of wellness. Stress wears on the daily physical and mental systems and processes that sustain us. Extended exposure to unmanaged stress can bring physical and mental problems that can literally be life threatening.

In a medical or biological context stress is a physical, mental, or emotional factor that causes bodily or mental tension. Stresses can be external from the environment, such as found in psychological, or social situations, or internal functions such as illness, exhaustion or a medical procedure. Stress can initiate the "fight or flight" response, a complex reaction of neurologic and endocrinologic systems.

It is the physical and emotional responses to stress that can create problems. Elevated heart rates, hypertension, secretions of compensating hormones such as Cortisol and other physiological reactions can cause damage to bodily systems over time. Continued and unresolved mental stress can lead to mental and emotional breakdown requiring expensive and time consuming treatment to remedy.

Your quiet place needs to be structured to allow daily stress to be de-escalated. You have to discover ways and methods of managing that stress and the stressors causing it. In your quiet place, integrating solutions that calm the body and mind and allow you to recover from stress is critical.

Obviously this implies that any quiet place you choose should be free from physical locational stressors. It also implies that your time in your quiet place should be productive in "unstringing your bow" to allow stress to be minimized. The methods to do this are as numerous as individuals looking for a calming influence. Reading, prayer, meditation uplifting music… whatever format your release valve might entail.

Your Quiet Place is for Healing also

Certain stressors will require more than just release. For deeper stressors, results of long term exposure or more pressing issues such as trauma or abuse, a process of healing needs to take place. Healing is more than just recovery. Healing is a permanent release from physical or psychological stressors that have plagued someone for an extended period of time. Many individuals carry scars from trauma in childhood or young adulthood that, if unaddressed, may create adverse reaction and continued stress throughout their lives.

Finding a quiet place means accurately identifying such stressors and cognitively taking steps to relieve them. This begins with a recognition that such stressors exist, and then tying them to the correct causes that created them. This is often not a process that can be undertaken alone. If the trauma causing stress is deep enough professional assistance is recommended. There are times that healing cannot begin without help getting to a point to accurately identify how that healing can specifically take place.

Be willing to seek healing and change when it is called for. There is great strength and personal power in casting aside burdens that should not be carried on and endless basis. Heal from the daily, grinding stress that can wear us all down. But seek to heal from larger, endemic burdens that may have been carried for years. You are the only one who can clearly identify what those burdens might be and decide to shed them. You deserve the release and renewal. You are worth it!

Quick Tips to Finding Your Quiet Place

- If you have the option to do so, transform a room with a new paint job, plants, a throw rug, warm lighting and a comfortable chair to create a space that speaks to you in a quiet, creativity-inducing way.
- Always have an "escape route" to a calming place within reach of your home and your work. If you are feeling over-stressed, spend a few minutes enjoying your private refuge.
- Identify libraries, reading rooms or other community areas where you can enjoy quiet and contemplative time without the intrusion of others.
- Learn a discipline of meditation and resolve to integrate periods of quiet meditation into your fitness routine.
- Treat yourself to a massage, wrap or other spa treatment that relaxes you completely. Share the experience with a friend or partner if possible.
- Participate in a retreat with others with a like-minded desire for healing from an internal stress. Discuss stressors or abuse that have worn on you over time. Actively exercise healing methods learned.
- Explore well documented behavioral interventions such as Cognitive Behavioral Therapy to relieve a carried trauma from earlier in life. Be proactive in the healing process.
- Find your favorite park, beach, mountain or forest trail. Visit your quiet place often. You have earned it.

APPENDIX I – FINANCIAL WELLNESS PRINCIPLES

A discussion of wellness would not be complete without discussing the basics of financial wellness. Financial wellness is compromised of two components, healthy financial management and productive vocational pursuits. The two components are obviously closely related. It is hard to manage finances if you are not earning sufficiently to support your basic needs. Conversely, even the highest professional earners can meet with disaster if they do not manage their earnings according to sound financial principles.

Sound financial management is worthy of an entire volume in itself. For the purpose of wellness we will break it down onto a few fundamental principles. Wider reading and study on the subject is strongly recommended. Our focus is to discuss those basic financial guidelines that will bring basic security and over which you have control.

Financial wellness exists in a background of economic wellness and prosperity. Economic environments expand and contract. While you should always have a finger on the pulse of your economic surroundings, you have no control over the macroeconomic developments that may impact your financial prosperity. The best you can do is to abide by time-tested practices and take advantage of the opportunities you encounter.

Like most other aspects of a modern world, financial management can be quite complex. But the basic underlying principles that can help you successfully manage finances and career decisions never change. It is these consistent guidelines that deserve your attention.

Seven Fundamental Financial Wellness Principles

1) Always Pay Yourself First:

The most common misconception in finance is that we work and earn in order to pay for a certain standard of living. It is the apartment or home, car, clothes, furnishings, and other accoutrements that are the goal of making money. This is a counterintuitive way of thinking. The first priority in working and earning, and the primary way to guarantee financial wellness is to pay yourself first. Pay yourself, in a manner that contributes to a long term goal of being eventually freed from the necessity to work on a daily basis in order to earn.

This is accomplished by setting aside a specific amount of each dollar earned into pre-tax and post tax savings vehicles that can accumulate interest and investment earnings over time. This includes standard savings or investment accounts, but also encompasses tax-deferred savings vehicles such as Regular or Roth Individual Retirement Accounts (IRA), 401(K) accounts, Simplified Employee Pension Plans and other legal vehicles.

You may set up your own savings vehicles such as an IRA or may be able to participate in an employer sponsored program such a company 401(K) plan. Take advantage of the opportunities the tax code provides to set aside and invest amounts each time you get paid. Allow those accounts to build, and over a period of years (the years that encompass your working career), with proper investment returns those monies will add up to a point you do not have to work any longer. This principle is applicable no matter how much you earn throughout your lifetime.

Discipline yourself to save by paying yourself first and learn to live off of the remaining income. It is foolish to spend every earned dollar on consumer goods. Those goods will not pay you back over time. Most assets other than real estate depreciate rapidly once purchased. Savings vehicles (in a normal economic market) appreciate over time.

It is possible for anyone who works and saves (by consistently paying themselves first) to reach a point of financial independence. And the quintessential definition of financial wellness is to be independent of any other party in terms of your own financial control. This can primarily be accomplished by paying yourself first and allowing remaining funds to accommodate normal living expenses.

2) Money In needs to Equal or Exceed Money Out:

After paying yourself first, the next most important principle is to be disciplined with budgetary spending. This means tracking dollars in and creating and maintaining a budget on dollars out. If you do not know where your money is going and on what it is being spent, you are not in control of your finances. If your finances are not in control, you cannot achieve financial wellness.

There are numerous ways to budget. Simple paper records, including receipts and payroll statements, can do the job if consistently maintained. There are numerous budgeting Apps and software solutions on the market. Many financial institutions will have online resources to help track spending and create budgets based on the income and outflow from your accounts.

The simple question is will you have the discipline to apply and use a budget? Just like the discipline and responsibility you must embrace to be active and well in other wellness principles, you should hold yourself accountable in knowing precisely how and why you spend.

3) Understand the Power of Money and Time:

If you will take the time to pay yourself first and remain disciplined in saving, the next principle to master is to understand clearly the power of compound growth of money over time. This is particularly applicable in tax-deferred savings where interest and investment return build without taxable consequences until taken out in later years as distributions.

At an ordinary return rate, every dollar saved turns into many dollars over a period of decades if invested well. This principle of compounding, where interest and investment returns build upon themselves over a long window of investment time, increases your net worth exponentially.

The wise use of interest and investment returns presupposes an understanding of the proper vehicles to yield these returns. This is a subject worthy of study. Also, there are numerous investment professionals that are eager to supply information and resources to make these investment decisions a reality.

Network in your local market with licensed professionals that can introduce you to a large universe of financial products and options. Study them carefully and learn of the concepts of risk and return and develop strategies that are tolerable for your personality and investment philosophy.

4) Distinguish Between Wants and Needs:

The world we live in is a consumer driven paradigm. The health of the American economy depends on high levels of consumerism. The messaging you receive from day to day is "buy, buy, buy". Unfortunately, satisfying unlimited consumer desires has little correlation with financial wellness. Particularly if obtaining consumer items might involve spending beyond a reasonable budget and taking on debt.

In a society being prodded incessantly towards instant gratification, it requires a specific discipline to step back and identify what you really need versus things you merely want. Consumer wants vary widely. It is well and fine to gratify yourself with some items that are pleasing and contribute to a wellness lifestyle. It is another thing altogether to consume endlessly and acquire more and more consumer goods.

Your concept of appropriate consumerism should be aligned with a healthy and well view of self. Do you allow your "things" to define you? Are you clear that the status of such things do not define who you really are? True wellness involves distinguishing those consumer items you need to provide a solid lifestyle versus things that become transformational to your self-vision.

Keep in mind that, at least from a perspective of wellness, possessions are merely items that contribute to your healthy lifestyle and/or allow you to be your best with yourself and with others. If intangible items take on a larger role than that, if you begin to define yourself based on the "wants" of your life, especially if you are using them to compare yourself with others, you are treading on thin ice. A material based perspective of self, despite significant achievement that may lead to material wealth, is an unsound foundation on which to define yourself. The truly well individual keeps these wants in their proper perspective.

5) Avoid Unnecessary Debt:

Excessive consumerism and consumer debt will create the opposite of financial wellness. Debt is bondage. Debt is an untiring and merciless master. Debt is a huge stressor and can destroy financial wellness and erode personal security and confidence. It is far better from a perspective of wellness to save and prepare fiscally to buy consumer goods (goods which have a short financial life as well as a finite service life) than to take on debt. Often, consumer debt will still be owed beyond the life of the product that was borrowed for.

Certain borrowing is necessary in a modern setting. Few people can pay cash for a house or new car. But perhaps a house that is the minimum necessary to house a family versus a larger luxury home and a slightly used car versus new creates less debt burden. Large debt burdens, especially those that can last for years or decades, can be a significant source of concern if not managed properly.

One sub-principle that should never be ignored is the idea of putting consumer debt onto a real estate loan that amortizes over fifteen to thirty years. If debt must be used for consumer goods, make sure that debt is paid off around the time the item has expired in its usefulness.

When and where to take on debt is also an important strategic decision. For example, moving from an apartment and purchasing a home should be a decision made when income and job prospects are stable and you expect to be in one location for at least three years. Purchasing a new car may or may not be wise when your current vehicle has middling mileage and runs well. Timing and circumstance must be taken into consideration when contemplating debt.

When it comes to revolving debt, such as credit card debt, plan to pay off those debts as soon as possible, preferably monthly. Revolving debt often a carries high interest rates and, if not paid quickly, can cause consumer items to cost several times their original price just from the interest paid on carrying that item. When it comes to wellness, debt is rarely your friend.

6) Prioritize and Plan:

Just as it is important to have a fitness plan to achieve the goals you envision, so a financial plan is wise for your various phases of life. In younger years, prime earning years and years approaching retirement there will be differing priorities. When it comes to meeting your needs and satisfying wants, a good plan will identify priorities there also.

As with other Pathways, an idea not quantified and put into writing is just a wish. Use available resource, including professional financial advice, to establish, follow and execute a sound financial plan for your life. It contributes highly to a well state of being to know what your financial pathway is, how far it goes, and where you are on that pathway.

Identify and set your priorities, plan and execute around those priorities and periodically evaluate and be honest with how you are doing.

7) More Money does not Equal More Satisfaction:

The old truism states that money cannot buy happiness. Or, as the Beatles used to sing, "Money can't buy me love". While studies have shown that having sufficient funds to manage a comfortable lifestyle creates less stress and more overall satisfaction, there is a point where money and lifestyle reach a point of diminishing return. In other words, when is enough genuinely enough?

Tremendous earnings do not guarantee long term satisfaction or even financial security. There is a long history of celebrities, professional athletes and others who have earned fantastic sums over a career and wound up penniless. Additionally, if the pursuit of additional income crowds out other considerations of wellness in your lifestyle, it can be detrimental. When it comes to financial wellness, sometimes quality of finances can be more important than quantity.

All of the money in the world may not be helpful if you have catastrophic health events. All of the career success imaginable may be wasted if you cannot enjoy the smaller and finer things in your life that would engender complete wellness. Often, obtaining tremendous wealth creates the need to manage that wealth or the resources producing wealth that consume every waking hour. Success can be addictive, and financial success equally so. You must consider how that will impact balance in other aspects of your life.

This is not to say that the pursuit of success is a negative. Quite the contrary. Pursuit of excellence, the type of excellence embraced by complete wellness, is a worthy and high standard. It simply implies that those pursuits should be placed in line with all of the other considerations that would comprise a lifestyle of complete wellness.

Career paths are more nebulous today than ever. Twenty five percent of jobs coming in the next decade do not even exist yet. A typical person working over forty years may change careers six or more times. Such is the rapid march of innovation and technology. To create secure wellness in your career path, also known as vocational wellness, you must be open to continuing your education and professional development. Career decisions are significant decisions, and time, study and sometimes a bit of luck will help.

The first guideline that applies is to know yourself and your strengths and weaknesses. Be honest where your skills are best. Are you a "people" person or a "numbers" person? Can you work in a stressful, fast paced environment or do you prefer steady and predictable? If you train and work to your strengths, you will obviously be more successful. If you continue to develop those strengths, adding professional knowledge and experience, you have a chance to rise to the top of your field. Consistent effort and development over time will yield benefits.

The second guideline is to always be open to continuing education and professional development. With rapidly moving technology comes the need for continual upgrading of knowledge and skills. Change in itself is stressful, but a commitment to focus on personal development within a given field will counter that stress and support vocational wellness. Again, if you are willing to give the time and effort you will generally harvest positive outcomes financially.

The third guideline is to recognize that experience is the most valuable teacher and you should always leverage your experience. Many employers today are placing experience over education. Many graduate programs will not accept students without several years of practical experience. Catalog your experiences. Create a spreadsheet of accomplishments and skills. Be proud of what you have done and envision what that experience has prepared to do next. Then find a creative way to let the people who should know discover your accomplishments.

Remember, financial wellness is about more than numbers and monetary success. It is about making the best of what you have and planning and utilizing those assets you acquire in an intelligent manner. Financial wellness follows the same pattern as physical wellness. You study, gather information, work and form a plan and execute that plan. If you follow these simple guidelines you are sure to enjoy financial success to some extent.

APPENDIX II – WELLNESS FROM THE HOME TO THE WORKPLACE

The recognition of the importance wellness has taken center stage over the last decade or so. Wellness integrated into a positive lifestyle has been well documented in bringing innumerable benefits not only to the individual, but in adding value to the community and employer alike. Wellness, approached correctly, changes lives and enhances the bottom lines of communities and corporations.

The institutional and social costs of disease need no elaboration. One catastrophic illness can wipe out a lifetime's worth of assets for an individual or family. One or two employees in need of major medical intervention can drive up health costs for everyone covered under an employer group benefit plan.

Wellness begins at home, with each and every individual. It starts with a fundamental daily recognition that proper lifestyle choices not only bring a fuller, richer and more complete life, but also create economic benefits as well. The best way to minimize the cost of illness or disease is to prevent that illness or disease in the first place.

Wellness can be a somewhat private and individual undertaking, but it can also be a group activity. When it comes to wellness, there is often strength in numbers. While the Twelve Pathways outlines suggestions for group activities to support individual efforts, there is a broader, more institutional level at which wellness can be proliferated.

This is known in common parlance as corporate or workplace wellness. Numerous companies, small and large, are now realizing the benefits of sponsoring wellness programs and interventions for their employees. There are two fundamental cases for sustaining a wellness program in the workplace. The first case revolves around the economic argument for wellness. The second encompasses the more subjective humanistic results wellness brings.

The Economic Argument for Workplace Wellness

When it comes to a cost benefit discussion of wellness, it is clear that for employers and employees alike the numbers add up. A Harvard study recently found that every dollar spent on a workplace wellness program resulted in nearly four dollars not spent on medical costs. Based on the fundamental programs and interventions surveyed that savings figure might greatly increase if broader and more comprehensive interventions were utilized. Whatever analysis you utilize, wellness brings economic benefit.

The current benefits model has been around for over fifty years. With regards to wellness, in terms of preventive care and methodology, it is outdated. Current health insurance models emphasize care after disease or illness has occurred. Outside of a regular physical, there is little provision for any paradigm of disease prevention. It simply is not addressed in any significant detail.

Traditional health insurance benefits are offered for full time employees, currently defined as anyone working over thirty hours per week, to provide a method of mitigating medical costs to that employee. There is usually a deductible and co-payment provision that varies depending on the plan. The cost of the plan is shared between employer and employee and can range from hundreds to thousands of dollars per month depending on the thoroughness of coverage.

While health insurance benefits are important for protecting and retaining employees, a comprehensive wellness program should be added to any benefits provision, or even provided in cases where no benefits are available. The case for this results from the fact that a properly structured and administered wellness program provides an economic backstop to numerous employee problems that can be caused by disease or illness. This is accomplished by tested strategies for disease prevention versus treatment after the fact.

The traditional benefits model provides benefits at a substantial premium, then pays for health costs incurred after a plan participant has become ill or needs to treat a medical condition. The dollars spent to heal or repair the problems of the individual contribute to an actuarial number known as benefits plan experience. Annual renewals are based on the plan utilization from the previous years and can average double digit increases.

The more prudent yet underutilized structure is to invest in wellness up front in addition to or in lieu of benefits dollars and prevent the individual from coming down with major illness or disease, thus saving both the company and the employee unnecessary cost and suffering. This should be the emerging thought among benefits and risk management professionals. The analysis flow is illustrated below:

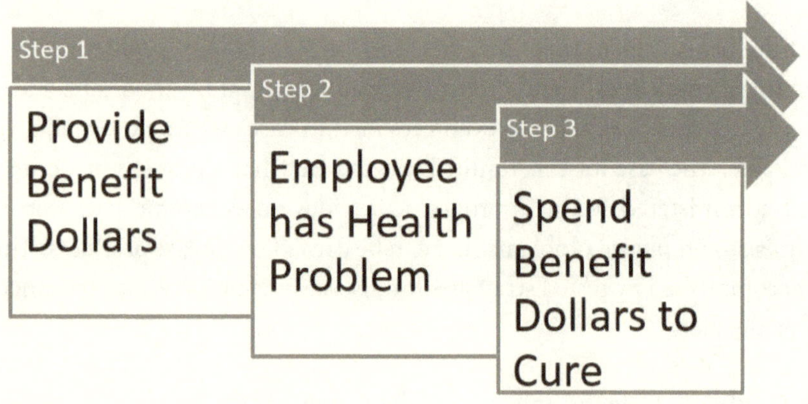

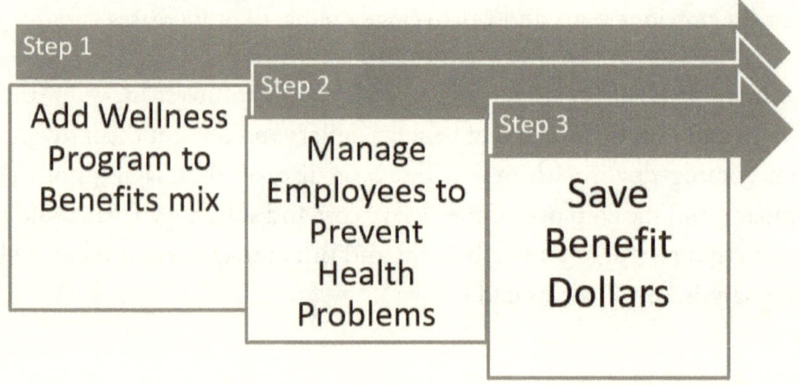

The economic argument for wellness centers on the saved costs for the employer as well as the savings to the employee in terms of shared health care costs. In fact, some studies show that with proper wellness management the average output is 81% less in incurred health care expenses for the average participant. That is a tremendous savings to both the company bottom line and the individual employee. It will reflect directly over time in reduced renewal costs.

Economic benefits do not stop with a reduction of health care expenses however. There are several other areas in which a properly administered wellness program can beneficially impact a company. These are less direct than health care cost savings but impact the company and employees in a positive manner nonetheless.

The first area of impact is in recruiting and retention. There are few better ways for a company to attract the best people and show that they care for their employees more than a vibrant wellness program. Done correctly, wellness communicates a distinct message that "our company cares about its employees". Wellness takes that message straight to the hearts and minds of everyone involved.

Wellness also increases on-the-job productivity while reducing absenteeism. Individuals who take on wellness as a lifestyle tend to have more energy, are sick less often, have clearer thought processes and show more initiative on the job. When you take pride in your overall wellness, you tend to take pride in other areas of your life. This is directly reflected in improved performance.

Recent research concluded that employees who take wellness seriously are 37% more productive than employees who do not have such standards. This is reflected in greater performance combined with less absenteeism. In addition, employees engaged in wellness show greater job satisfaction. That is a dynamic hard to measure in absolute dollars, but increased productivity, reduced turnover and satisfied employees are certainly goals of any quality employer.

The Subjective Case for Wellness in the Workplace

In addition to the economic arguments, wellness can be a significant driver of increased company culture, enforcing excellence throughout an organization using the principles of wellness as primary tools. In the classic works of organizational theory such as "In Search of Excellence", "Seven Habits of Highly Effective People" or Theory Z" there is a clear and compelling case for managing and refining the culture of any organization.

Wellness is, in essence, an investment in both the individual employee and the overall flavor and strength of a company's culture. With constant administration and care, wellness reflects a reinforcement of accurate, proper and caring attitudes within the organization. Wellness is based on correct principles of human dynamics. To enforce those principles on an organizational level is to simply emphasize what should be obvious. Yet that emphasis, as effective as it is, is often overlooked when considering the overall fabric and priorities of organizational culture.

Wellness on a group level has been shown to increase employee satisfaction. It engenders greater cooperation, communication and teamwork. It reinforces the impression of a positive work environment and places emphasis on care for each individual. In the larger context of organizational culture, these regular touchpoints of emphasis create a positive image over time.

This reinforcement becomes very real in the minds of each individual as they are encouraged to achieve their personal best in every area of their lives, both within and without the organization. Over time, these continual impressions are woven tightly into the fabric of the organization, driving culture upward with a continual positive and caring message. Wellness is a powerful tool in continually emphasizing excellence.

The Necessary Components of a Group Comprehensive Wellness Plan

For a well-managed wellness program to be effective in a workplace setting there are several components that are necessary. The goal of any wellness program is to affect change. Change in the lifestyle of each individual translates into broader change for the organization, along with all of the subjective and economic benefits mentioned.

The first and overwhelmingly most important component is a management commitment to the concepts of wellness. Without organizational leadership recognizing and supporting a culture of wellness, the details of a program may not matter. Top down support is critical. Management buy in should be more than just a strict bottom line equation. It should include a philosophical recognition of all the subjective benefits wellness can bring and a determination to integrate wellness into company culture and policy.

Along with that leadership support, the specific avenues of implementing wellness are equally important. The first element of infusing wellness into an organization revolves around offering an online platform rich with program resources that can be utilized regularly by employees. An online platform will contain places to record daily wellness performance data, create personal and group challenges, offer information on exercise programs, recipes, rewards, menus of activities and other wellness related subjects.

In companies that are large enough they may often assign an employee, often through human resources, to be an internal wellness coordinator of online platforms and programs. These functions can be done internally or in conjunction with a third party program provider. However it may be structured, the online platform leads to the next element which is a plan for continual employee engagement.

Vehicles for regular employee engagement are a critical component to an effective wellness program. A program not engaged in is not a program. It is an unfulfilled aspiration. Engagement can begin with the measurement and gathering of data. A standard vehicle for gathering initial data is known as a Personal Health Assessment. Any worthwhile platform will include this component, which is a self-directed questionnaire and data gathering of lifestyle choices and identifiable risk factors. In addition certain biometrics should be gathered on employees individually. This can be done by health professionals or a certified wellness coach.

Biometrics are clinical measurements of specific factors that can determine present and future health risks. Biometrics need to be regularly measured and monitored to be effective and produce information from which an individualized, effective, specific and targeted wellness program can be designed. Some basic biometrics include:

- Waist Circumference
- Waist to Hip Ratio

- Total Body Weight
- Body Mass index
- Body Fat Percentage
- Blood pressure
- Triglycerides
- HDL Cholesterol
- LDL Cholesterol
- Blood Glucose
- Hemoglobin A1C
- C Reactive Protein
- Cotinine Levels
- Bone Density
- Blood Oxygen Levels

The components listed are considered the minimum for a basic group wellness program. The underlying assumption of such programs is that individuals provided with such programs will be motivated self-starters in employing wellness into their lifestyle. Such programs "check the box" in terms of providing a wellness program, but do not necessarily create long term behavioral change.

These programs will give self-starters, those who find their own internal motivation to engage in wellness and can easily overcome entry barriers, attractive tools to explore. But they do not necessarily provide the impetus for other categories of participants. As with any such programs the participant population will consist of self-starters, fence sitters and avoiders.

Self-starters will quickly recognize the benefits of the program and engage in a majority of activities on their own volition. Fence sitters will watch the program, perhaps dabble in a few of the offerings and may or may not engage in a consistent manner. Fence sitters will also often engage initially, only to disengage shortly thereafter without an external source of motivation. Avoiders do exactly what their categorization implies. They avoid engaging in a program altogether.

Unfortunately, the self-starters are often the ones most fit to begin with. They see a wellness program as a helpful vehicle to move their own wellness levels upwards. It becomes endemic on the program sponsor to find ways to motivate the fence sitter and avoider. They are often the individuals most in need of behavioral change and mitigation of health risk factors. But they are also the type of individual that needs a helping hand, and external source of motivation

The transition from the basic program to a more comprehensive and effective program, a program that can engage fence sitters and avoiders, involves one additional crucial component. That component is a dedicated and well trained wellness coach. One on one, face to face coaching is the one aspect that can affect true change and sustain that change long term.

Such change comes from an additional layer of detail and accountability. A well trained and properly informed wellness coach can counsel directly with their individual clients and help them personalize programs based on health assessment and biometric data. Personal wellness plans, including diet, exercise routines and critical lifestyle changes can be designed, discussed and agreed upon by the coach and client. That role of reinforced guidance, or trusted counselor, defines the proper intervention and additional layer of accountability a coach can provide.

It should be generally accepted as true that you, and each and every individual, has the ability to determine what is best for themselves when it comes to wellness. The coaching component guides individuals into seeking, applying and ultimately holding themselves accountable for what constitutes that "best". A "return and report" system with a knowledgeable coach provides a sounding board and a specific time frame for implementing activities that will bring results. Coaches can offer an alternative perspective as to the veracity or effectiveness of certain activities or plans and bring additional professional information and interventions.

This is the component that engenders immediate and lasting change. The additional layer of accountability a wellness coach brings cannot be replicated in an online only intervention. The relationship of professionalism and trust a good coach brings encourages each individual to strive to improve. When a person can be taken by the hand and shown a clear path to better health, more energy, improved appearance and many other beneficial outcomes, they tend to discover their own internal motivation.

A proper plan, effectively communicated spurs behavioral change. The activities defined in that plan, faithfully and regularly executed bring results. Results reinforce the desired changes and begin to move an individual up the hierarchy of wellness perspective and attitude. Results change attitudes, attitudes changes lifestyle choices. Proper choices change lives. It all begins with creating that accountability. Results can change an avoider into a self-starter.

With each of the above outlined components in place, a comprehensive wellness culture can be created and maintained in almost any organization. That wellness centered culture will impact both the bottom line of a company and the personal lives of everyone who participates. Wellness works.

Wellness is the Future

There is a demographic problem across the modern postindustrial world. The birth rate, and subsequent replacement rate, has dropped precipitously over the last fifty years. Simply put, the nuclear family is changing and couples are not having children in near the numbers they once did. Replacement rates across the United States have dropped to around 1.7. This means for every two people that pass away, only 1.7 are being born. In Europe, that rate is critically low at around 1.4. The implications for future work forces and economies are significant.

As an employer, this directly translates to the fact that for every two people who retire, there is only a bit more than one and a half people coming down the pipeline to replace them. How is a company's work force, competitiveness and succession planning to be maintained? Where are the necessary new employees to come from? How will they be incented, trained and retained in a high demand market combined with shrinking human capital?

Some would argue that automation might pick up that slack. Perhaps in a few more production oriented professions that might be one solution. A more immediate answer would be the need to recruit and retain the best possible employees, either domestically or through importation. In this human resource strategy, wellness plays a powerful role. As prime employee pools shrink, the excellence of a company's culture in attracting the best and brightest in any given industry becomes more and more critical.

A wellness culture, combined with powerful and effective wellness programs, will go a long way in defining excellence in any given industry. No matter the business or the service, whatever outcome a company or industry can produce, wellness can improve on people and processes.

The idea of comprehensive wellness on a group level has arrived. It is simply a matter of education and implementation to allow the benefits of wellness to take root and reinforce change at an organizational level. As we demand more out of individual employees, and as the pool of qualified employees gradually contracts, wellness is a differentiator. Wellness works because the principles of wellness are constant and unchangeable. As long as we are human, wellness will make us better at who we are and what we do.

AFTERWORD

Over thirty years have passed since that fateful day in New Jersey. It has indeed been a long but fruitful journey. I would not change much over the years, at least as it relates to the internalization of personal wellness. If anything, I might learn to relax a bit more and not push so hard day in and day out. Wellness has brought a dimension and fullness to living I am sure I would not have known otherwise. There have been many wonderful activities and events, good friends and memorable times over the years directly attributable to a love of wellness and the activities that support it.

Running has turned out to be a primary enjoyment and a long history of road racing has created some of my fondest memories. From the Manufacturer's Hanover Corporate Challenge races in Manhattan to the State Olympics nestled in the heart of the Rockies, middle distance races have been a principal entrée in a years-long diet of fun and competitive activities. Age, time and wear and tear have slowed the mileage and required more diverse activities. Through this I have discovered many related pursuits that have provided great pleasure for me and my family. Hiking, biking, cross country and downhill skiing, golf and swimming have all had their supplemental roles to a steady diet of aerobic and resistance training.

There have been times of great life changes, times of great stress, long commutes to far away work places, the addition of children, sleep deprivation, injuries and a whole host of other obstacles to chip away at continued wellness. But through a consistent vision and careful planning I have been able to execute my goals rather succinctly throughout these many years. In the post-fifty world, doctors and regular physicals have become a more integrated part of the program, as are holistic supplementation and intervention.

In addition, I have committed the remainder of my career to bringing the numerous benefits of wellness to others. This is the fulfillment of a lifelong dream and I can think of few causes more worthy of time and effort. Wellness changes lives and it changes them for the better. Such pursuits hardly seem like work at times, it is more of a pleasure to share these great benefits.

Although wellness gives no guarantees of longer life, and cannot stop hair from eventually graying or skin from wrinkling, it improves the quality of life all along the way. It has taught me discipline and a mastery of self I doubt I would know otherwise. Wellness has shown me a pathway to living life to its fullest. If it has done it for me, it can do it for you also. All you have to do is understand and apply the basic principles found in the Twelve Pathways. I will be watching for you as we move purposefully down the road!

www.ingramcontent.com/pod-product-compliance
Lightning Source LLC
Chambersburg PA
CBHW051100250726
48656CB00001B/390